Adjunctive Technologies in the Management of Head and Neck Pathology

Editors

NAGI M. DEMIAN
MARK E. WONG

ORAL AND MAXILLOFACIAL SURGERY CLINICS OF NORTH AMERICA

www.oralmaxsurgery.theclinics.com

Consulting Editor
RICHARD H. HAUG

May 2014 • Volume 26 • Number 2

ELSEVIER

1600 John F. Kennedy Boulevard ● Suite 1800 ● Philadelphia, Pennsylvania, 19103-2899

http://www.oralmaxsurgery.theclinics.com

ORAL AND MAXILLOFACIAL SURGERY CLINICS OF NORTH AMERICA Volume 26, Number 2
May 2014 ISSN 1042-3699, ISBN-13: 978-0-323-29721-9

Editor: John Vassallo; j.vassallo@elsevier.com
Developmental Editor: Yonah Korngold

Oral and Maxillofacial Surgery Clinics of North America (ISSN 1042-3699) is published quarterly by Elsevier Inc., 360 Park Avenue South, New York, NY 10010-1710. Months of issue are February, May, August, and November. Business and Editorial Offices: 1600 John F. Kennedy Blvd., Suite 1800, Philadelphia, PA 19103-2899. Periodicals postage paid at New York, NY and additional mailing offices. Subscription prices are $385.00 per year for US individuals, $567.00 per year for US institutions, $175.00 per year for US students and residents, $455.00 per year for Canadian individuals, $680.00 per year for Canadian institutions, $520.00 per year for international individuals, $680.00 per year for international institutions and $235.00 per year for Canadian and foreign students/residents. To receive student/resident rate, orders must be accompanied by name or affiliated institution, date of term, and the *signature* of program/residency coordinator on institution letterhead. Orders will be billed at individual rate until proof of status is received. Foreign air speed delivery is included in all *Clinics* subscription prices. All prices are subject to change without notice. **POSTMASTER:** Send address changes to *Oral and Maxillofacial Surgery Clinics of North America,* Elsevier Periodicals Customer Service, 11830 Westline Industrial Drive, St. Louis, MO 63146. Tel: 1-800-654-2452 (U.S. and Canada); 314-447-8871 (outside U.S. and Canada). Fax: 314-447-8029. E-mail: journalscustomerservice-usa@elsevier.com (for print support); journalsonlinesupport-usa@elsevier.com (for online support).

Reprints. For copies of 100 or more, of articles in this publication, please contact the Commercial Reprints Department, Elsevier Inc., 360 Park Avenue South, New York, NY 10010-1710. Tel.: 212-633-3874; Fax: 212-633-3820; Email: reprints@elsevier.com.

Oral and Maxillofacial Surgery Clinics of North America is covered in *MEDLINE/PubMed* (*Index Medicus*), *Science Citation Index Expanded* (*SciSearch®*), *Journal Citation Reports/Science Edition*, and *Current Contents®/Clinical Medicine*.

Contributors

CONSULTING EDITOR

RICHARD H. HAUG, DDS
Carolinas Center for Oral Health, Charlotte,
North Carolina

EDITORS

NAGI M. DEMIAN, DDS, MD, FACS
Associate Professor, The University of Texas
School of Dentistry; Chief of Oral and
Maxillofacial Surgery Service, Oral &
Maxillofacial Surgery Department, Lyndon B.
Johnson Hospital; Director of The Externship
Program; Medical Director of the ACLS
Course, Dental Branch at UTHSC,
Houston, Texas

MARK E. WONG, DDS
Chairman and Program Director, Professor,
Department of Oral of Maxillofacial Surgery,
University of Texas Health Science Center at
Houston, The University of Texas Medical
School at Houston, The University of Texas
School of Dentistry at Houston, Houston,
Texas

AUTHORS

IBRAHIM ALAVA III, MD
Department of Otorhinolaryngology, University
of Texas Health Science Center at Houston,
Houston, Texas

JENNIFER ATLAS, MD
Fellow, Hematology and Oncology,
Comprehensive Cancer Center of Wake
Forest School of Medicine, Winston-Salem,
North Carolina

ANGEL BLANCO, MD
Memorial Hermann Hospital, Houston, Texas

ERIC R. CARLSON, DMD, MD, FACS
Professor and Kelly L. Krahwinkel Chairman,
Department of Oral and Maxillofacial Surgery;
Director of Oral and Maxillofacial Surgery
Residency Program; Director of Oral/Head and
Neck Oncologic Surgery Fellowship Program,
University of Tennessee Medical Center,
University of Tennessee Cancer Institute,
Knoxville, Tennessee

STEVE CHIANG, MD
Clinical Assistant Professor of Radiology, The
Methodist Hospital, Houston, Texas

NAGI M. DEMIAN, DDS, MD, FACS
Associate Professor, The University of Texas
School of Dentistry; Chief of Oral and
Maxillofacial Surgery Service, Oral &
Maxillofacial Surgery Department, Lyndon B.
Johnson Hospital; Director of The Externship
Program; Medical Director of the ACLS
Course, Dental Branch at UTHSC,
Houston, Texas

ERIC J. DIERKS, DMD, MD, FACS
Director of Head and Neck Oncologic
Surgery Fellowship; Attending Surgeon,
Trauma Service and Oral and Maxillofacial
Surgery Service, Legacy Emanuel Medical
Center; Affiliate Professor, Department
of Oral and Maxillofacial Surgery, Oregon
Health and Science University; Head
and Neck Surgical Associates, Portland,
Oregon

AHMED EID, MD
Assistant Professor General Oncology, The
University of Texas MD Anderson Cancer
Center, Houston, Texas

RODOLFO GARZA, DDS
Resident, Oral & Maxillofacial Surgery,
University of Texas Health Science Center
at Houston, Houston, Texas

ALLAN M. HENSLEE, PhD
Department of Bioengineering, Rice University,
Houston, Texas

F. KURTIS KASPER, PhD
Department of Bioengineering, Rice University,
Houston, Texas

IVAN L. KESSEL, MD
Associate Professor, Department of Radiation
Oncology, University of Texas Medical Branch,
Galveston, Texas

SHUANG LI, MD
Resident, Internal Medicine, University of
Texas Health Science Center at Houston,
Houston, Texas

**JAMES ANTHONY MCCAUL, PhD,
FRCS(OMFS), FRCS, FDSRCPS,
MBChB(Hons), BDS(Hons)**
Professor, Consultant Maxillofacial/Head and
Neck Surgeon, The Royal Marsden Hospital;
UK RCS/BAOMS/Saving Faces Maxillofacial
Surgery Specialty Lead for Research, London,
United Kingdom

ANTONIOS G. MIKOS, PhD
Department of Bioengineering, Rice University,
Houston, Texas

BENJAMIN J. SCHLOTT, DMD, MD
Fellow, Oral/Head and Neck Oncologic
Surgery, Department of Oral and Maxillofacial
Surgery, University of Tennessee Medical
Center, University of Tennessee Cancer
Institute, Knoxville, Tennessee

SARITA R. SHAH, BS
Department of Bioengineering, Rice University,
Houston, Texas

JONATHAN W. SHUM, DDS, MD
Assistant Professor, Department of Oral and
Maxillofacial Surgery, University of Texas
Health Science Center at Houston, Houston,
Texas

PATRICK P. SPICER, PhD
Department of Bioengineering, Rice University,
Houston, Texas

EMILIO P. SUPSUPIN Jr, MD
Department of Diagnostic and Interventional
Imaging, Houston Medical School, University
of Texas Health Science Center, Houston,
Texas

ALEXANDER M. TATARA, BS
Department of Bioengineering, Rice University,
Houston, Texas

NADARAJAH VIGNESWARAN, BDS, DMD
Director, Oral and Maxillofacial Pathology
Biopsy Service; Professor, The University of
Texas School of Dentistry at Houston,
Houston, Texas

Y. ETAN WEINSTOCK, MD, FACS
Department of Otorhinolaryngology, University
of Texas Health Science Center at Houston,
Houston, Texas

MICHELLE D. WILLIAMS, MD
Director, Surgical Pathology Fellowship
Program, Head & Neck Section, Department of
Pathology; Associate Professor, UT MD
Anderson Cancer Center, Houston, Texas

MARK E. WONG, DDS
Chairman and Program Director, Professor,
Department of Oral of Maxillofacial Surgery,
University of Texas Health Science Center at
Houston, The University of Texas Medical
School at Houston, The University of Texas
School of Dentistry at Houston, Houston,
Texas

Contents

Head and neck squamous cell carcinoma is the sixth most common cancer world-wide predominately associated with tobacco use. Changing cause and increased incidence in oropharyngeal carcinomas is associated with high-risk types of human papilloma virus and has an improved survival. Optical devices may augment visual oral examination; however, their lack of specificity still warrants tissue evaluation/biopsy. Histologic factors of oral carcinomas are critical for patient management and prognostic determination. Clinical biomarkers are still needed to improve early detection, predict malignant transformation, and optimize therapies.

The success of mandibular reconstructions depends not only on restoring the form and function of lost bone but also on the preservation of the overlying soft tissue layer. In this case study, 5 porous polymethylmethacrylate space maintainers fabricated via patient-specific molds were implanted initially to maintain the vitality of the overlying oral mucosa during staged mandibular reconstructions. Three of the 5 patients healed well; the other 2 patients developed dehiscences, likely due to a thin layer of soft tissue overlying the implant. The results presented provide evidence that a larger investigation of space maintainers fabricated using this method is warranted.

Accurate assessment of surgical margins in the head and neck is a challenge. Multiple factors may lead to inaccurate margin assessment such as tissue shrinkage, nonstandardized nomenclature, anatomic constraints, and complex three dimensional specimen orientation. Excision method and standard histologic processing techniques may obscure distance measurements from the tumor front to the normal tissue edge. Arbitrary definitions of what constitutes a "close" margin do not consider the prognostic significance of resection dimensions. In this article we review some common pitfalls in determining margin status in head and neck resection specimens as well as highlight newer techniques of molecular margin assessment.

Surgery is the primary intervention in oral and maxillofacial tumors and under ideal circumstances is curative. There is no evidence to support the use of induction or adjuvant chemotherapy in initial therapy of early stage tumors. Locally advanced tumors, non-resectable tumors as well as recurrence in early stage disease, need a multi-modality therapeutic approach involving chemotherapy. Palliative chemotherapy plays an important role in the treatment patients with metastatic oral and maxillofacial tumors. Chemotherapy and targeted agents plays an important role in the treatment of patients with rare oral and maxillofacial tumors such as sarcomas, lymphomas, and giant cell tumors.

Osteonecrosis of the jaws associated with bisphosphonate and other anti-resorptive medications (ARONJ) has historically been a poorly understood disease process in terms of its pathophysiology, prevention and treatment since it was originally described in 2003. In association with its original discovery 11 years ago, non-evidence based speculation of these issues have been published in the international literature and are currently being challenged. A critical analysis of cancer patients with ARONJ, for example, reveals that their osteonecrosis is nearly identical to that of cancer patients who are naive to anti-resorptive medications. In addition, osteonecrosis of the jaws is not unique to patients exposed to anti-resorptive medications, but is also seen in patients with osteomyelitis and other pathologic processes of the jaws. This article represents a review of facts forgotten, questions answered, and lessons learned in general regarding osteonecrosis of the jaws.

Oral health care in patients undergoing chemotherapy and/or radiation therapy can be complex. Care delivered by a multidisciplinary approach is timely and streamlines the allocation of resources to provide prompt care and to attain favorable outcomes. A hospital dentist, oral and maxillofacial surgeon, and a maxillofacial prosthodontist must be involved early to prevent avoidable oral complications. Prevention and thorough preparation are vital before the start of chemotherapy and radiation therapy. Oral complications must be addressed immediately and, even with the best management, can cause delays and interruption in treatment, with serious consequences for the outcome and prognosis.

This article presents an overview of the evaluation and staging of the neck in the context of malignant disease. The current tumor-nodes-metastasis (TNM) nodal classification is reviewed followed by a brief discussion of the common malignant processes encountered in the head and neck and their associated risk factors for cervical metastasis. Common imaging modalities, such as ultrasound, magnetic resonance imaging, computed tomography, and positron emission tomography, for the investigation of the neck are also summarized.

Radiation therapy (RT) is an important modality in the treatment of head and neck cancers. Significant morbidity can result, however, because of exposure of normal tissues to high doses of RT. Advances in planning and delivery, especially intensity modulated radiation therapy, can reduce the risk of these toxicities by ensuring that the tumor and draining lymph nodes are adequately treated, while the surrounding organs and tissues at risk are avoided. Image guidance during treatment delivery allows for smaller margins around the tumor to account for variations in daily setup and positioning. All these advances help to improve the quality of life of cancer survivors.

ORAL AND MAXILLOFACIAL SURGERY CLINICS OF NORTH AMERICA

RELATED INTEREST

Otolarnygologic Clinics of North America
August 2013 (Vol. 46, No. 4)
Oral Cavity and Oropharyngeal Cancer
Jeffrey N. Myers and Erich M. Sturgis, *Editors*

THE CLINICS ARE NOW AVAILABLE ONLINE!
Access your subscription at:
www.theclinics.com

Preface
Adjunctive Technologies in the Management of Head and Neck Pathology

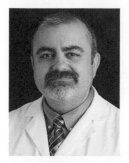
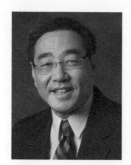

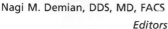

Nagi M. Demian, DDS, MD, FACS Mark E. Wong, DDS

Editors

The management of head and neck pathology is an ever-evolving discipline and the diagnostic and treatment modalities Involved are as varied as the taxonomy of the different diseases included. The purpose of this issue of the *Oral and Maxillofacial Surgery Clinics of North America* is not to provide a comprehensive review of pathology but to describe some of the adjunctive therapies and measures used in the management of these conditions. Several disciplines participate in the treatment of head and neck pathology and we have received contributions from the major participants. While the management of pathology and head and neck malignancy may not be a principal focus for many oral and maxillofacial surgeons, extensive opportunities exist to care for these patients, and familiarity with current treatment approaches is necessary. Topics representing new and dynamic treatments, such as the management of necrosis of bone secondary to antiresorptive therapy, and others that oral and maxillofacial surgeons may not be familiar with, such as chemoradiation therapy for cancer patients, were included. Although an exhaustive review of head and neck pathology was never the goal or within the scope of this publication, efforts were made to make this edition a practical and useful review of some of the more significant developments in the management of head and neck pathology.

The editors thank our participating authors, many of whom are clinical collaborators. Their contributions stand as a testimony to the importance of multidisciplinary collaborations in the treatment of patients with head and neck pathology.

Nagi M. Demian, DDS, MD, FACS
Oral & Maxillofacial Surgery Department
Oral and Maxillofacial Surgery Service
Lyndon B. Johnson Hospital
Houston, TX, USA

Dental Branch at UTHSC
UT Annex 112 B
5656 Kelly Street
Houston, TX 77026, USA

Mark E. Wong, DDS
Oral & Maxillofacial Surgery
University of Texas Health Science Center at
Houston
6516 MD Anderson Boulevard
Houston, TX 77030, USA

E-mail addresses:
nagi.demian@uth.tmc.edu (N.M. Demian)
mark.e.wong@uth.tmc.edu (M.E. Wong)

Oral Maxillofacial Surg Clin N Am 26 (2014) ix
http://dx.doi.org/10.1016/j.coms.2014.03.001
1042-3699/14/$ – see front matter © 2014 Elsevier Inc. All rights reserved.

Epidemiologic Trends in Head and Neck Cancer and Aids in Diagnosis

Nadarajah Vigneswaran, BDS, DMD[a],*,
Michelle D. Williams, MD[b]

KEYWORDS

- Epidemiologic trends • Head and neck cancer • Diagnosis • Squamous cell carcinomas

KEY POINTS

- Head and neck squamous cell carcinoma is the sixth most common cancer worldwide predominately associated with tobacco use.
- Changing causes and increased incidence in oropharyngeal carcinomas are associated with high-risk types of human papillomavirus and have an improved survival.
- Potentially malignant disorders include a range of entities that vary from low to extremely high risk of transformation to carcinoma as seen in proliferative verrucous leukoplakia.
- Optical devices may augment visual oral examination; however, their lack of specificity still warrants tissue evaluation and biopsy.
- Histologic factors of oral carcinomas are critical for patient management and prognostic determination, including depth of tumor invasion, perineural invasion, margin status, presence of regional lymph node metastases, and presence of extracapsular extension within metastases.
- Clinical biomarkers are still needed to improve early detection, predict malignant transformation, and optimize therapies.

CHANGING EPIDEMIOLOGY OF HEAD AND NECK CANCER

Incidence

Head and neck cancers represent the sixth most common cancer worldwide, with approximately 630,000 new patients diagnosed annually resulting in more than 350,000 deaths every year.[1] More than 90% of head and neck cancers are squamous cell carcinoma (HNSCC) that arise from the mucosal surfaces of the oral cavity (OSCC; International Classification of Diseases, Tenth Revision [ICD-10] code C00-08), oropharynx (OPSCC; ICD-10 code C09-10 and C12-14), and larynx (ICD-10 code C32-9). Although in Northern America and Europe HNSCC accounts for 5% to 10% of all new cancer cases, there is wide geographic variation in the incidence and anatomic distribution of HNSCC worldwide. This variation is predominately attributed to demographic differences in the habits of tobacco use and alcohol consumption, which contribute to the development of almost 80% of all HNSCCs diagnosed globally. In high-risk countries (ie, India, Sri Lanka, Bangladesh, and Pakistan), OSCC is the most common cancer in men and the third most common cancer in women.[2] Among the European countries, the highest incidence of OSCC is in

Disclosures: This work was supported by Cancer Prevention Research Institute of Texas (CPRIT) grants # RP101382 & RP100932.

[a] Oral and Maxillofacial Pathology Biopsy Service, The University of Texas School of Dentistry at Houston, 1941 East Road BBSB, Room 5320, Houston, TX 77054, USA; [b] Surgical Pathology Fellowship Program, Head & Neck Section, Department of Pathology, UT MD Anderson Cancer Center, 1515 Holcombe Boulevard, Unit #085, Houston, TX 77030, USA

* Corresponding author.

E-mail address: nadarajah.vigneswaran@uth.tmc.edu

Oral Maxillofacial Surg Clin N Am 26 (2014) 123–141
http://dx.doi.org/10.1016/j.coms.2014.01.001

France, with high rates also noted in Hungary, Slovakia, and Slovenia.[2] In the United States, HNSCC constitutes only the eighth most common cancer among men, with approximately 53,600 patients diagnosed yearly, and shows a considerably lower mortality with 11,500 patient deaths annually.[3] The decreasing incidence of OSCC and laryngeal SCC in the United States and in other developed countries coincides with a decline in the use of tobacco products.[4] By contrast, there is a recent upsurge in the incidence of OPSCC, which is attributed to a change in the biologic driver of SCC in this region, with an increasing frequency of an association with high-risk subtypes of human papilloma virus (HPV).[4,5] HPV-associated SCC involves specific anatomic sites, specifically the oropharynx, which includes the base (posterior one-third) of the tongue, tonsils, and the lateral pharyngeal walls (oropharynx), coinciding with the Waldeyer ring of lymphoid tissue to include the nasopharynx.[6] Conversely, HNSCCs involving the anterior two-thirds of the tongue (oral tongue), floor of the mouth, palate, buccal mucosa, sulcus, and gingiva are considered HPV-unrelated sites. Importantly, in the 1980s, only 16% of carcinomas in the oropharynx in the United States were HPV-positive, whereas now more than 75% of OPSCC is HPV-positive.[7] Indeed, HPV-driven HNSCC is responsible for a more than 25% increase in the incidence of HNSCC in the United States during this past decade, primarily among middle-aged men.[6] Currently, the incidence of HPV-related HNSCC in the United States is 6.2 per 100,000 and 1.4 per 100,000, for males and females, respectively.[7] Currently, HPV-related OPSCC is recognized as a distinct subset of HNSCC because of its unique cause, molecular pathogenesis, clinical presentation, and therapeutic responses, which are discussed in detail later in this article.

RISK FACTORS FOR HNSCC
Tobacco, Alcohol, Pan

The risk for developing HNSCC is associated with several factors, including geographic location, habits, diet, and genetic background. Among all etiologic factors, cigarette smoking and excessive consumption of alcohol represent the most important risk factors for the development of HNSCC and have a synergistic effect.[8] Cigar and pipe smoking also increase the risk for developing OSCC, with pipe smokers having a predilection for lower lip SCC. Reverse smoking, a habit practiced in certain areas of India and South America, in which the lighted end of the cigarette is kept inside the mouth while smoking, causes HNSCC involving the hard palate. Chewing of the betel quid (also known as *pan*) is linked to the development of HNSCC of the buccal mucosa and the mandibular buccal sulcus. The habit of betel quid chewing is highly prevalent in countries with the highest incidence of OSCC (ie, India, Pakistan, Bangladesh, and Sri Lanka). The betel quid consists of betel leaf, areca nut, and slaked lime with or without added tobacco. Tobacco and areca nut are the 2 important carcinogens that are linked to the devolvement of OSCC. The relative risk for OSCC was 7.74 for betel quid with tobacco, whereas the relative risk reduces to 2.56 for betel quid without tobacco.[9] The use of smokeless tobacco in the form of loose-leaf chewing tobacco, moist or dry snuff (finely ground tobacco), or chewing tobacco, a habit prevalent in the United States and Scandinavia (ie, Sweden), is linked to OSCC with predilection in the mandibular buccal sulcus and gingiva. The relative risk for OSCC associated with chewing tobacco and moist snuff is quite low, ranging from 0.6 to 1.7, whereas the use of dry snuff is associated with a higher relative risk, ranging from 4 to 13.[10] Although alcohol is not considered to be a carcinogen, excessive alcohol intake increases the risk of HNSCC, most often acting synergistically with tobacco.[8,11]

HPV

One-fifth of HNSCC cases currently diagnosed in the United States are not related to cigarette smoking and/or alcohol abuse. Infection with high-risk HPV types (HPV 16, 18, 31, and 33) plays a causal role in the pathogenesis of OPSCC with distinct clinical and molecular features (**Table 1**). Specifically, HPV high-risk type 16 accounts for more than 90% of HPV-associated OPSCC in the United States, with rare accounts of HPV type 18, 33 and others reported in the literature.[12] The shift in biology to HPV over tobacco-associated SCC also accounts for the improvement in overall survival seen in patients with HNSCC.[6] HPV is a strong prognostic factor. For SCC treated with similar therapeutic interventions (predominately radiation therapy with or without chemotherapy), HPV-associated SCC showed an 82% 3-year survival compared with 57% survival for smokers with SCC.[13] This survival difference continues at 5 years. However, when patients have both an HPV+ tumor and a strong tobacco exposure, the prognosis of these patients may not parallel HPV+ tumors exclusively. To date, how HPV and smoking status should be used to potentially alter therapy remains debated and under investigation in clinical trials.

Table 1
Comparison of conventional/tobacco-associated SCC and HPV-associated SCC

	HPV-Associated SCC	SCC (Conventional/Tobacco Exposure)
Age (mean y)	53	57
Sex	M>F 2.8:1.0	M>F 1.5:1.0
Location	Tonsils, base of tongue>>nasopharynx	Oral cavity, larynx
LN	30%–60% present at initial presentation Often cystic LN metastases Maybe bilateral	Prognostic factor
Prognosis (disease-specific survival)		
3 y	82%	57%
Morphology	Often nonkeratinizing High nuclear-to-cytoplasmic ratio Relatively monotonous	Usually keratinizing Surface dysplasia may be seen
Associated with	HPV types 16>>18>others	Tobacco exposure
Molecular alterations	High overexpressed p16[a] (IHC) Blocked Rb, p53 by viral E6, E7 HPV +high-risk types 16>others	LOH in Chr 3p and/or Chr 9p and others Mutated p53

Abbreviations: Chr, Chromosome; F, female; IHC, immunohistochemical evaluation; LN, lymph node metastases; LOH, loss of heterozygosity; M, male.
[a] p16 overexpression is not always associated with HPV status, particularly outside of the oropharynx.

Other Contributing Factors

Chronic sun exposure and associated ultraviolet light radiation are linked to the development of SCCs of the lips. Other less known risk factors for HNSCC include iatrogenic immunosuppression for solid organ or bone marrow transplant, family history of HNSCC, consuming diets deficient in antioxidants, and older age.[2]

DISEASES AND SYNDROMES ASSOCIATED WITH INCREASED RISK FOR HNSCC
Plummer-Vinson

An increased risk for HNSCC is seen in patients with Plummer-Vinson syndrome that is characterized by iron deficiency anemia, atrophic glossitis, and esophageal webs. Plummer-Vinson syndrome frequently affects middle-aged women and is rarely encountered in the United States.

Fanconi Anemia and Dyskeratosis Congenita

Fanconi anemia (FA; Mendelian Inheritance in Man (MIM) 227650) and dyskeratosis congenita (DC; MIM 30500,127550, 224230) are 2 hereditary cancer syndromes that predispose to HNSCC at an early age. FA is a chromosomal instability disorder inherited as an autosomal- or X-chromosomal recessive trait caused by germline mutations in one of 15 FA genes involved in the DNA repair

pathway resulting in increased risks for bone marrow failure, leukemia, and solid malignancies.[14] HNSCC is the most frequently diagnosed solid cancer in patients with FA. The risk of HNSCC among patients with FA is 800-fold higher than in the general population and occurs at a younger age (median age: 27 years) than the general population.[15,16] Frequent oral screening in patients with FA for premalignant lesions is essential to try and reduce morbidity from OSCC. Similar to FA, DC is also an inherited bone marrow failure disorder that is caused by defects in telomere maintenance.[17] HNSCC is the most common solid malignancy seen in patients with DC. The oral cavity is the predominant site for HNSCC in both patients with FA and patients with DC, frequently occurring in the tongue.[18] Hence, semiannual oral cancer screenings are recommended for both patients with FA and patients with DC, beginning at a very young age.

AGE, SEX, AND RACE PREDILECTION OF HNSCC

Similar to other cancers, the risk of developing HNSCC also increases with age, and most HNSCC occurs in patients age 50 or older. The average age for a smoking-related HNSCC diagnosis is 60 years (median age: 63 years), whereas the average age for smokeless tobacco–related

HNSCC is 78 years.[19] HPV-related HNSCC is usually diagnosed at younger ages than tobacco-related HNSCC.[20] The median age at diagnosis of HPV-related HNSCC is 58 for men and 61 for women.[20] HNSCC is more common in men than in women, and the ratios of OSCC and OPSCC by sex are currently about 1.5:1.0 and 2.8:1.0, respectively. In the United States, African-American men have a higher incidence of conventional tobacco-related HNSCC than Caucasian men. In contrast, HPV-related HNSCCs are more frequently diagnosed in Caucasian men.[20]

ANATOMIC SITES OF HNSCC
Tongue

Anatomic sites of HNSCC exhibit significant geographic and demographic variation because of differences in their cause. In the United States, the oral tongue is the most common intraoral site of HNSCC, with 7100 new cases diagnosed annually, and accounts for 25% to 40% of all OSCC.[21,22] The incidence of OSCC of the tongue has been steadily increasing from 1975, whereas the incidence of other OSCC sites has been decreasing.[23–25] Furthermore, recent studies report an increased incidence of oral tongue carcinomas arising in young white women who are more likely to have never been smokers and or drinkers.[23,26] Oral tongue carcinomas occurring in young patients without the traditional risk factors of tobacco and/or alcohol abuse exhibit a more aggressive clinical course characterized by higher rates of locoregional recurrences, shorter disease-free intervals, and poor survival, all without a known etiologic cause.[23,27] Carcinoma of the oral tongue is the most aggressive of all OSCCs and exhibits extremely high rates of occult lymph node metastases (not detected by clinical and radiographic imaging studies).[28] Histopathologic guidelines used for the management of occult neck metastasis for early-stage tongue SCC are described later.

Floor of Mouth

The floor of the mouth is the second most common (15%–20%) intraoral site for SCC, followed by the gingiva, accounting for 10% of all OSCC. In the United States, OSCC rarely occurs in the dorsal surface of the tongue, hard palate, and buccal mucosa. SCC of the lip occurs in light-skinned individuals, and more than 90% of lip SCCs are located on the lower lip. Lip SCCs are considered distinct from intraoral carcinomas because of the differences in the cause and pathogenesis of these tumors.

PRECURSOR LESIONS OF HNSCC

Similar to other solid malignancies, HNSCC development is a multistep process, often with precursors, which are commonly known as precancerous or premalignant lesions. The expert Working Group of the World Health Organization Collaborating Center for Oral Cancer and Precancer on the terminology, definitions, and classification recently recommended the use of the term potentially malignant disorders (PMD), which includes premalignant lesions and conditions that have increased risk for malignant transformation.[29]

Premalignant Lesion

This lesion is a morphologically altered oral mucosal lesion in which HNSCC is more likely to occur than in its normal counterpart.

Premalignant Condition

This condition is a generalized state of the oral cavity, which is associated with a substantially increased risk for HNSCC.

Leukoplakia, erythroplakia, and palatal lesions in reverse smokers are considered precancerous lesions, whereas actinic keratosis, oral submucous fibrosis, and lichen planus are designated as precancerous conditions.[29] Tobacco- and alcohol-related HNSCCs are often preceded by lesions that present clinically as white (leukoplakia) or red (erythroplakia) patches or plaques. Currently, there are no known precursor lesions for HPV-associated oropharyngeal cancer.[30]

LEUKOPLAKIA

Leukoplakia is the most common and best-known form of PMD, accounting for 85% of all oral premalignant lesions. Leukoplakia is defined as a white patch or plaque that cannot be rubbed off and cannot be characterized clinically or histopathologically to any specific disease (**Fig. 1**). Hereditary, reactive, infectious, and immune-mediated disorders, which present as intraoral white patches or plaques resembling leukoplakia, are listed in **Table 2** (**Fig. 2**). The risk of malignant transformation of leukoplakias varies markedly and is dependent on

- Cause (smoking and/or alcohol use versus idiopathic)
- Clinical appearance
- Location
- Dysplasia grade on tissue biopsy

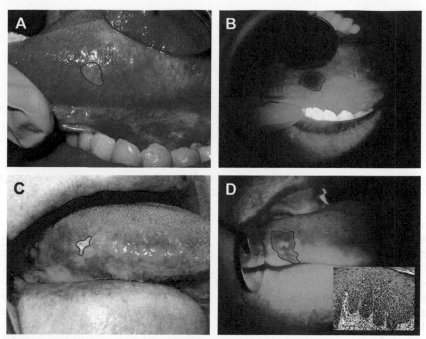

Fig. 1. Autofluorescence visualization of tongue leukoplakias. (*A*) A 57-year-old woman with a history of cigarette smoking presented with a leukoplakia that is barely visible under white light. (*B*) Autofluorescence visualization revealed loss of fluorescence of this leukoplakia. Excisional biopsy of this leukoplakia revealed moderate epithelial dysplasia. (*C*) A 65-year-old woman with no history of tobacco use presented with a leukoplakia in her lateral surface of the tongue. Extent of the leukoplakia involvement is markedly different when examined under white light (*C*) compared with autofluorescence visualization (*D*). Incisional biopsy of the lesion revealed moderate epithelial dysplasia (*inset*; [Hematoxylin and eosin (H&E) stain, original magnification ×100]).

In rare cases, patients may present with leukoplakia without any known etiologic factors, which is designated as idiopathic leukoplakia. Idiopathic leukoplakias have a significantly increased risk of malignant transformation than leukoplakias that are associated with a specific etiologic factor (ie, tobacco use).[31]

Leukoplakias most frequently occur at a single site (localized leukoplakia), are more common in men, and are associated with smoking. Localized leukoplakias presenting at a single site have 2 distinct clinical forms, namely, homogenous and nonhomogenous types, which are classified based on their surface color and appearance. Homogenous leukoplakias are uniformly white flat (patch) or slightly raised (plaque) lesions and exhibit a low malignant transformation risk. Nonhomogenous leukoplakias have a verrucous/granular surface, with or without red zones (speckled leukoplakia or erythroleukoplakia), and have a

Table 2
Clinical differential diagnoses for intraoral white patches and plaques

Localized Reactive and Infectious Disorders	Hereditary Diseases	Systemic Diseases
Frictional keratosis/benign alveolar ridge keratosis	Leukoedema	Lichen planus/lichenoid hypersensitivity reaction
Dentifrice-associated desquamation	Hereditary benign intraepithelial dyskeratosis	AIDS-oral hairy leukoplakia
Nicotine stomatitis	White sponge nevus	Lupus erythematosus
Smokeless tobacco keratosis	Dyskeratosis congenita	
Submucous fibrosis		
Hyperplastic candidiasis/candidal leukoplakia		
Leukoplakia		

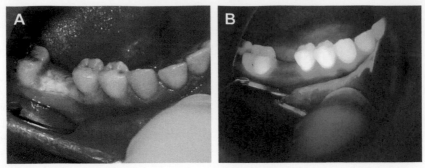

Fig. 2. Benign alveolar ridge keratosis that resembles leukoplakia is noted in a 49-year-old woman (*A*). Autofluorescence visualization revealed no loss of fluorescence (*B*).

higher risk for malignant transformation than homogenous leukoplakias. The intraoral site of the leukoplakia is the most important factor in determining its malignant transformation risk. In the United States and other Western countries, leukoplakias in the floor of the mouth, soft palate, and lateral/ventral surfaces of the tongue have the highest risk for malignant transformation. Overall, 9% to 37% of leukoplakias are expected to show dysplasia, carcinoma in situ, or invasive carcinoma at the time of biopsy.

Proliferative Verrucous Leukoplakia

A multifocal, proliferative and progressive form of leukoplakia is recognized as proliferative verrucous leukoplakia (PVL) (**Fig. 3**). PVL commonly

begins as a simple keratosis that eventually becomes verrucous and multifocal, involving large contiguous sites.[32] PVL is more common in elderly women, frequently involves the gingiva, and is not associated with either smoking or alcohol abuse (see **Fig. 3**). PVL tends to be persistent and frequently recurs even after surgical removal. PVLs are high-risk lesions, as almost 60% to 100% evolve into carcinoma over 10 to 20 years. Moreover, PVL generally lacks specific morphologic features, including the classic microscopic features of epithelial dysplasia, making PVL specifically a clinical diagnosis. Clinically and microscopically, PVL may mimic the plaque variant of lichen planus because of its multifocal involvement and frequent presentation of lichenoid inflammation in the biopsy.[33]

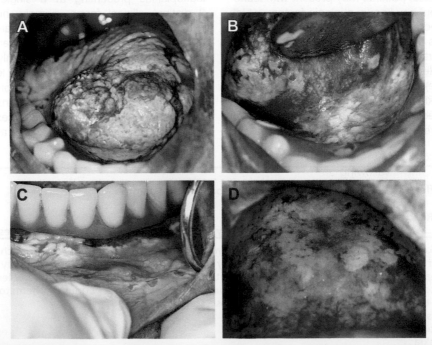

Fig. 3. Proliferative leukoplakia in an 82-year-old woman with no history of tobacco use. Initial biopsy performed 10 years ago was diagnosed as lichen planus. Multifocal PVL involves dorsal (*A*) and ventral (*B*) surfaces of the tongue, lip (*C*) and palate (*D*).

Erythroplakia

Erythroplakia is a less common form of a precancerous lesion or carcinoma that presents as a well-defined red, raised, velvety plaque that cannot be characterized clinically as any other disease. Oral mucosal conditions that may clinically resemble erythroplakia are listed in **Table 3**. Erythroplakias frequently occur in older adults in the floor of the mouth, ventral tongue, and soft palate. Frequently, erythroplakias are associated with adjacent leukoplakias (erythroleukoplakia). When biopsying these lesions, it is important to take the biopsy from the erythroplakic areas. Erythroplakias, unlike leukoplakias, are high-risk premalignant lesions because almost all erythroplakias (100%) will exhibit microscopically either dysplasia or in situ/invasive SCC at the time of biopsy. It should be emphasized that *leukoplakia* and *erythroplakia* are strictly clinical terms and are not associated with any specific histology and require biopsy for definitive classification.

Oral Submucous Fibrosis

Oral submucous fibrosis is considered a premalignant condition that is more prevalent among the South Asian population, and its incidence is highest in the Indian subcontinent. Oral submucous fibrosis is a chronic, progressive condition characterized by diffuse mucosal rigidity caused by dense fibrosis within the lamina propria that might extend into the underlying skeletal muscle. It is caused by chewing betel quid containing areca nut. The extent and severity of this disorder depend on the amount of areca nut in the betel quid and the duration and frequency of this habit. Oral submucous fibrosis frequently involves the buccal mucosa, tongue, and soft palate. The affected mucosal surfaces appear pale, blanching, and marblelike with focal areas of atrophy and erythema (**Fig. 4**). Patients commonly present with trismus, burning sensation, and xerostomia; difficulties in speech, mastication, and swallowing are experienced at the advanced stages. Oral submucous fibrosis is a premalignant condition with a malignant transformation rate of 8% to 12% over the period of 10 to 15 years.[34]

Oral Lichen Planus

Lichen planus is the most common chronic autoimmune inflammatory disorder of oral mucosa, that affecting 1% to 2% of the adults in middle age. It is more common among women and tends to have multifocal lesions, often bilateral and symmetric in distribution. It frequently involves buccal mucosa, gingiva, and the tongue (**Fig. 5**). Based on the clinical presentation, the following clinical variants of lichen planus are recognized:

- *Reticular variant (classic pattern)*: White striations and/or papules, asymptomatic, occur frequently in the buccal mucosa;
- *Plaque variant*: Thick, white plaque clinically resembling leukoplakia, asymptomatic, occurs frequently on the dorsal surface of the tongue
- *Erythematous/erosive variant*: Diffuse red areas with focal areas of mucosal erosions and atrophy, painful, and frequently occurs in the gingiva (desquamative gingivitis);
- *Ulcerative/bullous variant*: Diffuse red-and-white patches with a central, chronic, non-healing ulcer frequently seen on the lateral and ventral surfaces of the tongue and buccal mucosa

The malignant potential of oral lichen planus has been controversial in the past; however, it is now considered to have a low malignant transformation rate of 1% over a 5-year period.[35] Oral epithelial dysplasias (OED) (lichenoid dysplasia) may exhibit a chronic inflammatory cell infiltrate consisting of mostly lymphocytes that resemble the chronic inflammation seen in lichen planus; however, OED has accompanying epithelial cellular alterations consistent with dysplasia as noted in **Table 4**.[36,37] Moreover, the plaque variant of lichen planus and PVL may also share similar clinical and microscopic features, leading to a misdiagnosis of lichen planus.[32]

Table 3
Clinical differential diagnoses for intraoral red patches and plaque

Localized Reactive and Infectious Disorders	Neoplastic/Others	Systemic Diseases
Erythematous (atrophic) candidiasis	Hemangioma	Atrophic lichen planus
Allergic (contact) mucositis	Kaposi's sarcoma-plaque stage	Lupus erythematosus
Erythema migrans (migratory glossitis)	Telangiectasia	Mucous membrane
	Purpura	pemphigoid

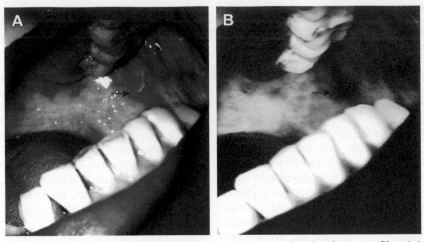

Fig. 4. A 52-year-old man with a history of betel quid chewing presented with submucous fibrosis involving bilateral buccal mucosa (*A*). Autofluorescence visualization showed enhanced fluorescence of the affected mucosa except for the erythematous area (*arrow*) revealing loss of fluorescence (*B*). An incisional biopsy taken from the area with the loss of fluorescence (*arrow*) revealed the presence of superficially invasive SCC.

AUTOFLUORESCENCE TISSUE-IMAGING DEVICES FOR SCREENING OF HNSCC AND ITS PRECURSORS

Early detection by screening and subsequent diagnosis of PMD is critical to prevent the onset of HNSCC, thereby decreasing morbidity and improving survival and quality of life. The current method for the screening of HNSCC and its precursors is clinical oral examination (COE), which consists of visual inspection and palpation of oral mucosa under white light. Several studies have shown that COE has limited value in detecting and distinguishing benign oral mucosal lesions that mimic HNSCC and its precursors (see **Fig. 1**).[38] Optical screening aids based on tissue reflectance and autofluorescence are increasingly used as adjuncts for COE for the early detection of oral premalignancies (**Box 1**). Detailed descriptions of the light-based screening devices for

PMD and their efficacy and limitations are reviewed elsewhere.[39,40]

Tissue autofluorescence imaging devices that are commercially available as adjuncts for conventional oral examination include VELscope (LED Dental Inc, White Rock, BC, Canada), Identafi 3000 (DentalEZ group, Malvern, PA), and OralID (OralID, Houston, TX). These optical devices use a special light source to illuminate oral mucosal surfaces with either blue/violet light (VELscope; 400–460 nM) or blue light (Identify and OralID; 405 nM). Oral epithelium and stroma absorb high-energy photons (short wavelength, 400–460 nM visible light) for excitation and emit a green (VELscope) (see **Fig. 1**) or blue (Identafi 3000 and OralID) (see **Fig. 4**) fluorescence spectra at longer wavelengths. The examiner can directly view the autofluorescence emitted by the normal tissue with the use of a long pass to block the reflected light. Epithelial fluorescence is produced by the

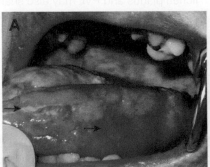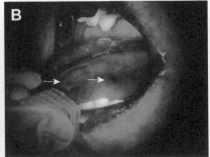

Fig. 5. Ulcerative form of lichen planus involving the tongue of 57-year-old woman (*A*). Autofluorescence visualization demonstrates loss of fluorescence limited to the erythematous areas (*arrows*) caused by inflammation (*B*).

Table 4
Effects of tissue changes in autofluorescence

Tissue Diagnosis[a]	Autofluorescence
Epithelial hyperplasia	No change
Dysplasia	Complete or partial loss
Invasive carcinoma	Complete loss
Verruciform hyperkeratosis (ie, PVL)	No change or increase
Inflammation	Complete or partial loss
Increased vascularity or vascular tumor	Complete or partial loss
Extensive fibrosis (ie, submucous fibrosis)	Increased
Exogenous pigmented lesion (ie, amalgam tattoo)	Complete loss
Endogenous pigmented lesion (ie, focal melanosis)	Complete loss
Surface bacterial or fungal colonization (ie, hairy tongue or candidiasis)	Altered red to orange fluorescence (porphyrin-related)

[a] Diagnosis as confirmed by tissue biopsy.

reduced form of nicotinamide adenine dinucleotide, flavin adenine dinucleotide, and keratin, whereas stromal florescence is primarily derived from collagen fibers with cross-links and elastin.

Box 1
Screening and diagnosis of PMD

Screening: evaluation of asymptomatic patients for presence of PMD

Gold standard: COE by an expert clinician

Adjunctive screening aids

- Transepithelial brush biopsy (ie, OralCDx Brush Test; OralCDx, Suffern, NY)
- Optical devices based on tissue reflectance visualization (ie, ViziLite Plus [ZILA Inc, Fort Collins, CO] & Microlux/DL [AdDent, Inc, Danbury, CT])
- Optical devices based on tissue autofluorescence visualization (ie, VELscope [LED Dental Inc, White Rock, BC, Canada], Identafi 3000 [DentalEZ group, Malvern, PA], and OralID [OralID, Houston, TX])

Diagnosis: a test performed in symptomatic patients to determine the diagnosis and treatment

Gold standard: scalpel biopsy for histopathologic examination

Adjunctive predictive tests[a]

- Loss of heterozygosity analysis
- TP53 mutational analysis
- DNA aneuploidy

[a] Currently, these tests are not routinely done in clinical practice but used for research application only.

Tissue autofluorescence emission can be affected by absorption and scattering of the excitation light by oxyhemoglobin and deoxyhemoglobin and enlarged and crowded cellular nuclei. PMD display loss of autofluorescence caused by altered metabolic activity and altered cellular and tissue architecture and appears dark brown or black, compared to adjacent healthy tissue with blue or green fluorescence (see **Figs. 1** and **4**). Tissue autofluorescence imaging is a valuable method to identify PMD with subtle mucosal changes or those that appear clinically occult under white light examination (see **Fig. 1**A, B). Fluorescence visualization is also very useful for discerning the extent of a lesion's involvement, selecting optimal biopsy sites, and aiding intraoperative surgical margins (see **Fig. 1**C, D). Tissue autofluorescence imaging is more effective than conventional oral examination in finding suspicious oral mucosal lesions; however, it demonstrates a low specificity in discriminating high-risk PMD from low-risk lesions because of the higher rate of false positivity associated with benign inflammatory/ulcerative oral mucosal lesions (see **Fig. 5**). Understanding how tissue factors alter the fluorescence spectra and related limitations of this technology are critical for proper use of tissue autofluorescence imaging devices in clinical practice (see **Table 4**).

ORAL EPITHELIAL DYSPLASIA

PMDs need to undergo a scalpel biopsy for microscopic diagnosis that will dictate their malignant transformation risk and the appropriate therapeutic management. Microscopically, these lesions may demonstrate epithelial hyperkeratosis, hyperplasia with or without dysplasia, carcinoma in situ, or invasive SCC (**Table 5**). As OED is a microscopic diagnosis of precancer without a specific clinical appearance, this term should not be used as a clinical description. Pathologically the term *epithelial atypia* is not synonymous with OED, and use should be restricted to epithelial changes not meeting the definition of dysplasia. An example of epithelial atypia is reactive and regenerative epithelial changes associated with inflammation adjacent to an ulcer. Hence, the use of the term *epithelial atypia* as a microscopic diagnosis for PMD may lead to confusion and should be avoided.

Both cytologic and architectural alterations of the oral squamous epithelium are taken into account when grading OED (see **Table 5**). However, microscopic evaluation of these features is subjective, which leads to significant interobserver and intraobserver variations in the diagnosis and grading of OED. The malignant transformation rate of OED varies considerably, ranging from 6% to 50% (mild dysplasia: 0%–5%; moderate dysplasia: 3%–15%; severe dysplasia: 7%–50%).[41] It should be noted that a significant proportion of cases that were diagnosed as benign hyperkeratoses without dysplasia have progressed to cancer. This outcome may be attributed to underdiagnosing clinical PVL secondary to the lack of specific cytologic features associated with dysplasia.

Although pathologic classification of OED is not an optimal criterion for predicting the malignant transformation risk of PMD, histologic grading of OED remains the gold standard to determine prognosis and to make treatment recommendations for these lesions. Currently, there are no reliable and reproducible molecular or genetic biomarkers that are superior to the diagnosis alone of OED in predicting malignant transformation risks to carcinoma. Although p53 mutations, loss of heterozygosity (LOH), and DNA ploidy analysis have been reported to predict the malignant transformation risk of PMD, none of these techniques have been adopted in the clinical practice.[42] LOH at chromosomes 3p and/or 9p increases the malignant transformation risk of OEDs by 22.6-fold compared with dysplastic lesions with 3p and 9p retention. OEDs with additional LOH on chromosomes arms 4q and 17p reveal a 41.7-fold increased risk for malignant transformation.[43]

Currently, there is no general consensus regarding the management of OED because of its variable biologic behavior, and grading of dysplasia is not the best predictor of its malignant transformation risk.[44] Moreover, interobserver and intraobserver variability in grading of dysplasia is another confounding factor impacting treatment decisions. The conventional management of OED is based on the dysplasia grade, clinical

Table 5
Histopathologic grading of OED

Grade	Cytologic Aberrations	Architectural Aberrations	Level of Involvement
Hyperkeratosis & hyperplasia	None	Hyperkeratosis, parakeratosis, or orthokeratosis Epithelial hyperplasia	Not applicable
Mild dysplasia	Increased nuclear/cytoplasmic ratio, nuclear hyperchromatism, & increased number of mitotic figures	Basal cell hyperplasia & sharply demarcated hyperkeratosis	Lower one-third of the epithelium
Moderate dysplasia	All of the above + variations in nuclear & cell size and shape, nuclear hyperchromatism, increased & abnormal mitotic figures	All of the above + loss of polarity & stratification, increased cell density with discohesion, bulbous or drop-shaped rete pegs	Lower half of the epithelium
Severe dysplasia	All of the above + mitotic figures within the superficial epithelial layers, increased number and size of nucleoli & apoptotic bodies	All of the above + dyskeratosis or keratin pearl formation	Lower two-thirds of the epithelium
Carcinoma in situ	All of the above	All of the above	Full-thickness epithelium

appearance, and the location of the lesion. Strategies used in the management of dysplasia include careful follow-up, surgical resection, cryotherapy, laser treatment, photodynamic therapy, and nonsurgical pharmacotherapy.[44] Complete surgical excision is the most commonly practiced approach for treating clinically evident premalignant lesions with moderate to severe dysplasia.[45,46]

Mild OED can be treated with either surgery or observation, depending on the location and clinical appearance of the lesion. Although surgical excision is the most effective method for preventing the recurrence and progression to invasive cancer, it is not always possible, especially in patients with OED who have widespread multifocal sites of involvement (ie, PVL). Surgical excision of these lesions is associated with significant functional and cosmetic impairments. Patients with multifocal or widespread OED should be closely monitored and rebiopsied if there are significant changes in their clinical appearance. Laser ablation and cryotherapy are alternative methods for treating OED with widespread involvement.[47] The major drawback of these treatments is that the tissue biopsy cannot be procured for histologic examination. If OED is to be treated with laser ablation, multiple representative biopsies of the OED should be taken for histopathologic diagnosis before commencing ablation. Cryosurgery with liquid nitrogen uses extreme cold to destroy dysplastic cells and is not widely used for treating OED because of the higher incidence of malignant transformation in patients with OED treated with cryosurgery compared with patients treated with surgery alone.[48] A new therapeutic approach for treating OED is photodynamic therapy, which involves the topical or systemic administration of a photosensitizing agent (ie, aminolevulinic acid) that when activated by light causes cytotoxic cell death by producing reactive oxygen species.[49] Randomized controlled trials are required to determine the effectiveness of photodynamic therapy in treating OED. Several clinical trials have tested various therapeutic agents for treating OED, and the relating data have been less impressive in preventing the malignant transformation of OED.

A recently published phase 1b study reported a 63% histologic response rate in OED when treated with a combination of erlotinib, an inhibitor of epithelial growth factor receptor (EGFR) and cyclooxygenase-2 inhibitor (celecoxib).[50] The data of this phase1b study seem promising, but additional clinical studies are needed before adopting this treatment strategy in routine clinical practice. There is currently no evidence-based, nonsurgical pharmacotherapy for managing OED.

PREDICTION OF PROGNOSIS, TREATMENT RESPONSE, AND SURVIVAL IN HEAD AND NECK CANCER
Biopsy Evaluation

Often, mucosal biopsies are superficial, curl/retract on removal, and may be tangential on sectioning. On histologic review, the determination of invasion may be limited or inconclusive secondary to scant underlying stroma and tissue orientation. Additionally, as a biopsy only accounts for one sampled area of the lesion, the pathologic interpretation must be correlated to the clinical findings for proper patient triage, and a higher-grade process cannot be excluded within the lesion. Thus a pathology reading of SCC at least in situ requires clinical correlation regarding the degree of suspicion for an invasive tumor, and this pathologic reading may represent a limitation of any superficial biopsy sample. Communication with the pathologist and possible rebiopsy should be considered when the clinical impression is discordant with the pathologic reading.

Rendering a diagnosis of SCC on a biopsy allows for further treatment planning; however, most of the prognostic factors rely on the evaluation of the resection specimen and the extent of disease. Specifically, pathologic factors in the primary tumor requiring evaluation include the grade of differentiation or histologic subtypes, depth of invasion, perineural invasion, and margin status, which all carry potential significance in determining the prognosis in HNSCC. Similarly, pathologic factors in regional metastasis including extracapsular spread impacts patient survival.

Histologic Subtypes of SCC

Conventional/keratinizing SCC
Conventional/keratinizing SCC represents the vast majority (80%) of squamous carcinomas in the head and neck outside of the oropharynx and nasopharynx. Conventional SCCs are graded based on both the extent of keratinization and cytologic maturation, as well as the growth pattern, into well, moderately, and poorly differentiated. This morphology is most often associated with tobacco- and/or alcohol-related HNSCC.

HPV-associated SCC (HPV+ OPSCC)
HPV-associated SCC (HPV+ OPSCC) morphologically is often more monotonous, with limited keratinization compared with conventional HNSCC (**Fig. 6**A). Terms including nonkeratinizing and basaloid have been confusingly used for HPV-associated SCC. Because the use of these terms is not referring to the specific subtypes of SCC typically associated with these descriptors,

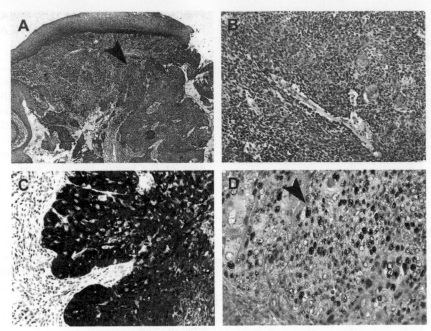

Fig. 6. HPV-associated SCC. (*A*) Low-power view (H&E, original magnification ×40) of the tumor arising in the tonsillar cryptic mucosa (*arrowhead*) deep to the surface mucosa. (*B*) Higher-power view (H&E, original magnification ×200) of monotonous, nonkeratinizing neoplastic cells typical of this phenotype. (*C*) Strong/overexpressed p16 immunohistochemical staining throughout the tumor (original magnifcation ×200). (*D*) HPV-positive in situ hybridization staining of the tumor nuclei (*arrowhead*) (original magnification ×200).

nonkeratinizing SCC of the nasopharynx and ba-saloid SCC, respectively, these terms should be avoided in this context. The distinct morphologic feature of HPV+ OPSCC also applies to lymph node metastases from these tumors. The lymph node metastases are often largely cystic by imag-ing and on histology, leading to the false associa-tion with branchial cleft cysts/carcinomas. Cystic neck masses in an adult must be fully evaluated, and metastatic SCC with cystic features is the leading diagnosis. Several less frequent subtypes of SCC are compared in **Table 6** and outlined later, each with its own challenges for diagnosis, partic-ularly on small biopsies.

Verrucous carcinoma
Verrucous carcinoma is a locally aggressive carci-noma showing a broad pushing growth downward and an exophytic/warty appearance (**Fig. 7**A). Cytologically, the cells are bland with minimal alteration (see **Fig. 7**A). Moderate dysplasia and thin, angulated rete ridges should raise a concern for a hybrid or conventional SCC. This distinction is important, as pure forms of verrucous carci-nomas do not metastasize; however, hybrid ver-rucous carcinomas with conventional SCC require consideration for local and regional eva-luation and treatment. Distinction on small bi-opsies may not be possible with the differential

including verrucous hyperplasia, which only shows an exophytic component and is more localized. Complete excision of these lesions with normal adjacent mucosa allows for definitive classification and treatment of these lesions.

Papillary squamous carcinoma
Papillary squamous carcinoma is infrequently encountered in the oral cavity with greater propen-sity for the nasal cavity and larynx. Biopsies show long papillary fronds lined by neoplastic cells without keratinization, overlying a fibrovascular core (see **Fig. 7**B). The exophytic growth pattern makes determination of invasion limited on bi-opsies secondary to scant underlying stroma. Thus, a pathology reading of SCC at least in situ with papillary growth requires clinical correlation regarding the degree of suspicion for an invasion tumor and often represents a limitation of a biopsy sample secondary to its superficial nature.

Basaloid squamous carcinoma
Basaloid squamous carcinoma is a distinct high-grade histologic variant of SCC, which morpholog-ically overlaps with solid adenoid cystic carcinoma and neuroendocrine carcinoma, requiring immu-nohistochemical evaluation to support final classi-fication in the absence of abrupt keratinization (see **Fig. 7**C). Basaloid SCC may be associated with

Table 6
Comparison of histologic subtypes of SCC

	Verrucous Carcinoma	Hybrid Verrucous/Conventional SCC	Basaloid Squamous Carcinoma	Papillary Squamous Carcinoma	Sarcomatoid Carcinoma
Age	Seventh–eighth decades	—	Seventh–eighth decades	Older	Seventh decade
Sex	M>F	—	M>F	M>F	M (smoking)
Location	Buccal, gingiva	—	Base of tongue, hypopharynx	Rare oral (larynx, sinonasal)	Larynx>oral/tongue
LN mets	None (if pure)	Risk for LN mets	High risk for mets	May metastasize	May metastasize
Gross appearance	Exophytic, warty, fungating	Exophytic	Variable/ulcerated	Exophytic- fronds, friable	Often polypoid, ulcerated
Morphology	• Abundant keratosis • Well differentiated • Minimal-atypia • Broad base, pushing border	• Mixture of verrucous & invasive SCC • Increased pleomorphism/dysplasia • Infiltrating border	• Immature basal-like cells • High N/C ratio • Rare abrupt keratin pearls • Mitoses • Central necrosis • Grows in nests & cords, cribriform, palisading • May have prominent basement membrane	• Full-thickness neoplastic cells • Without keratinization • Long fibrovascular cores • Biopsies often equivocal for invasion • Invasive nests looks like SCC	• Usually spindled • Low to moderate cellularity • Mitoses present • +/– Atypical mitoses • May see conventional SCC component • May show nearby dysplasia
Differential diagnosis	• Verrucous hyperplasia • WDSCC	• Verrucous hyperplasia	• Solid (basaloid) adenoid cystic carcinoma • Neuroendocrine CA	• In situ SCC	• Pseudosarcomatous inflammatory reaction • Sarcoma

Abbreviations: CA, carcinoma; F, females; LN, lymph nodes; M, males; mets, metastases; N/C, nuclear to cytoplasmic; WDSCC, well-differentiated SCC.

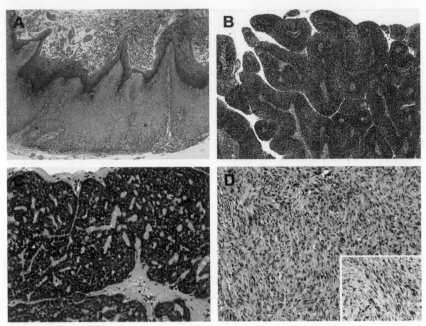

Fig. 7. Histologic variants of SCC. (*A*) Verrucous carcinoma showing a broad base, minimal cytologic atypia, and exophytic spire growth (H&E stain, original magnification ×40). (*B*) Papillary squamous carcinoma showing exophytic growth of fibrovascular cores covered by full-thickness neoplastic cells without keratinization (H&E stain, original magnification ×40). (*C*) Basaloid squamous carcinoma with high-grade features and scant cytoplasm often lacking keratinization as in this example (H&E stain, original magnification ×100). (*D*) Sarcomatoid (spindle cell) carcinoma haphazardly growing in sheets with pleomorphism and mitoses (H&E stain, original magnification ×100), often retaining cytokeratin expression detected by immunohistochemical staining (*inset* [original magnification ×100]), which aids in differentiating from true sarcomas.

HPV when this specific subtype arises in the oropharynx; however, basaloid SCC arising in other anatomic sites are HPV negative.[51] Information is still limited regarding the clinical significance of HPV+ in basaloid SCC and if this cohort also portends an improved survival as seen in other HPV-associated SCC in the oropharynx.

Sarcomatoid squamous carcinoma (spindled cell carcinoma)

Sarcomatoid squamous carcinoma (spindled cell carcinoma) is a high-grade tumor growing in sheets, often composed of pleomorphic spindled-shaped cells showing frequent mitoses, and may grow as an exophytic/polypoid mass (see **Fig. 7**D). Morphologically, this tumor overlaps with true sarcomas; however, sarcomas represent only a small minority of primary tumors in the head and neck region. Associated dysplasia or a history of prior dysplasia is also helpful in supporting the diagnosis of sarcomatoid squamous carcinoma. Ancillary testing with cytokeratins by immunohistochemical staining are often positive supporting the mucosal origin and the diagnosis of sarcomatoid carcinoma. Biologically, the transformation from a conventional SCC to a sarcomatoid SCC is thought to represent epithelial mesenchymal

transformation, with loss of adhesion molecules and gain of mesenchymal markers and invasive properties.[52]

HISTOPATHOLOGY PROGNOSTICATORS IN SCC

Histologic grading of SCC into well, moderate, and poorly differentiated carcinomas is based on the degree of keratinization and cytologic maturation resembling background squamous mucosa. Histologic grading of SCC remains of limited prognostic value, though it shows a trend for increased lymph node metastases in higher-grade tumors. In comparison, perineural invasion, as well as close margins (≤5 mm) and positive margin status, have shown a direct association with increased risk of local recurrence and tumor aggressiveness that may warrant adjuvant radiation therapy to achieve optimal local control.[53] Additionally, even early-stage tumors (T1), with clinically/radiographically N0 necks have a risk for occult metastases.[54] In primary SCC of the oral tongue and floor of the mouth, the best predictor of risk for regional metastases is the tumor depth of invasion, when radiographically the nodes are negative (cN0). At a depth of 4 mm or more in an oral tongue SCC, the risk of occult metastasis has been reported as high as 40% and is considered a sufficient risk to warrant a prophylactic neck dissection in this cohort of patients; moreover, a recent study suggests 3 mm or more as a better break point in oral tongue SCC for prophylactic neck dissection.[55,56] Similarly, a tumor thickness of more than 1.5 mm in the floor of the mouth region portends a higher risk for occult nodal metastases favoring prophylactic neck dissection (**Table 7**).[57] Tumor invasion into muscle shows similar correlation with an increased risk for regional metastases.[58] Other histologic factors, including tumor invasive patterns and associated tumor inflammation, may also allow for future risk classification and are currently undergoing prospective validation.[59]

Margins

Adequacy of margins must account for multiple anatomic and tumor parameters and is not simply black-and-white/positive or negative. Studies evaluating treatment failure/local recurrence and margin status in OSCC have demonstrated that even when a tumor is not at the margin, being close increases the risk for recurrence.[60] The definition of *close margin*, which would warrant consideration for additional tissue resection or adjuvant therapy, remains variable; however, the best consensus is 5 mm or more from the tumor for defining an adequate margin

in HNSCC.[60] Positive margins are considered SCC in situ or invasive tumor transected at the margin tissue edge. Additional considerations when studying distance to margins has been the marked shrinkage and retraction of tissue, particularly in tongue resections from the in situ distance measured by a surgeon from tumor to tissue margin, versus the ex vivo pathology measurement. Explanations for local failure with close surgical margins include perineural invasion, lymphovascular invasion, and small tumor nests infiltrating beyond the tumor mass with intervening normal stroma. Moreover, molecular studies on histologically negative margins have shown a wide range of molecular alterations (LOH, p53, and so forth), including known alterations associated with malignant progression.[61] The observation of precancerous molecular alterations also emphasizes the idea of field effect of precancerous changes in the oral cavity associated with tobacco exposure. Field cancerization increases the risk for both local recurrence and the development of second primaries.[60]

Lymph Node Metastases and Extracapsular Extension

In HNSCC, the most significant histologic prognostic factor for overall survival remains the presence of a positive lymph node metastasis, followed by the presence of extracapsular extension (ECE) of the tumor outside of a lymph

---

Table 7
Risk of occult metastases in oral SCC considerations for elective neck dissections

Study Population		Risk	Author/Conclusion
Stage I/II clinically N0		*Risk of recurrence*	
	• Elective neck dissection	1/28 pN0, 1/8 pN+	Yuen et al (71 patients)
	• Observation (no neck dissection)	11/35 (31%)	Elective neck dissection identified 22% occult LN mets and reduced risk of recurrence
Clinically T1/T2 N0	*Tumor depth of invasion*	*Risk of occult metastases*	
Tongue	<3 mm	1 of 23 (4.3%)	Zhang et al (65 patients)
	≥3 mm	13 of 42 (31%)	Recc neck dissection when an oral tongue SCC has a depth of invasion ≥3 mm
Tongue	<4 mm	0 of 14 (0%)	Sparano et al (45 patients)
	≥4 mm	13 of 18 (41%)	Recc neck dissection when an oral tongue SCC has a depth of invasion ≥4 mm
FOM	≤1.5 mm	1 of 57 (2%)	Mohit-Tabatabai et al (84 patients)
	1.6–3.5 mm	4 of 12 (33%)	Favors neck dissection for floor of
	>3.5 mm	9 of 15 (60%)	mouth SCC >1.5 mm in thickness

Abbreviations: FOM, floor of mouth; Recc, recommendation.

node.[62,63] Although most of the data are from oral SCC, the presence of ECE is now widely recognized as an adverse feature, including in other tumor types, which warrants consideration for intensified treatment regiments.[64] Survival data have shown more than a 4-fold increase in distant metastases and in death rates compared with node-negative patients. The most recent TNM tumor staging breaks ECE in lymph nodes into clinical/radiographic or macroscopic ECE versus pathologic microscopic ECE; this finding to date does not alter the overall staging of patients with HNSCC.

TUMOR STAGING

Unified systems for tumor staging (TNM) have allowed for more consistent use within the oral cavity and lip, though overall staging of tumors arising in the oropharynx remains distinct.[65] These sites begin with tumor size for T staging: Tis, is in situ; T1 are tumors up to 2 cm in greatest dimension; and T2 are more than 2 cm but less than 4 cm; T3 and T4 tumors are based on the extent of invasion into adjacent structures based on primary tumor site. N staging for the oral cavity and oropharynx is the same and is based on the metastasis size ($\leq$3, >3–6, and >6 cm greatest dimension), number of lymph nodes (single vs multiple), and location (bilateral, contralateral) of the lymph nodes relative to the primary. The overall staging combining the pathologic T and N score differs in oral cavity versus oropharynx primaries with allowable lymph node positivity in stage II OPSCC.[65] This system reflects the biologic distinctions of SCC based on the site of origin and the improved survival of patients with OPSCC compared with patients with OSCC.

DIAGNOSTICALLY RELEVANT IMMUNOHISTOCHEMICAL STAINS FOR HEAD AND NECK PATHOLOGY
Immunohistochemistry

The diagnosis of SCC is based on morphology and rarely requires ancillary studies for support of mucosal origin. However, in small biopsies, particularly of high-grade tumors, confirmation of carcinoma and derivation as squamous origin are required. Immunohistochemistry uses antibodies specific to proteins (keratins in carcinoma, S100 and melanin in melanomas, CD45 in lymphomas, and so forth) allowing for visualization of molecular expression under a light microscope. HNSCC typically express squamous epithelial marker cytokeratins 5/6 and p63, a basal cell/stem cell-like marker, is also often diffusely positive. The work-up of high-grade basaloid tumors includes cytokeratin positivity (negative in lymphomas and melanomas), p63 (positivity in SCC, negative in solid adenoid cystic carcinomas), and neuroendocrine markers (synaptophysin, chromogranin), which would be negative in SCC and positive in neuroendocrine carcinomas, small cell carcinomas, and Merkel cell carcinomas. Differentiating salivary tumors is performed primarily by their histologic pattern; however, salivary tumor cells are positive for cytokeratin 7 and may show intracellular mucin (mucicarmine special stain).

Makers for Infections

When evaluating tissue for infectious causes, special stains may be used to highlight the microorganisms. Grocott methenamine silver stain (GMS) is most widely used to highlight the wall of fungal organisms, with cultures advised for speciation. Periodic-acid-Schiff is frequently used to detect yeast and pseudohyphae (ie, candida) in tissue sections. Although gram stain highlights gram-positive and gram-negative bacteria, the high level of background oral flora makes this test less useful in the oral cavity. Actinomyces may form clusters visualized on morphologic review and are also highlighted by GMS and gram stains, though hematoxylin and eosin identification is sufficient to report the finding.

PROGNOSTIC BIOMARKERS FOR HNSCC
HPV and p16

Currently, only HPV and p16 testing are routinely performed as prognostic biomarkers in HNSCC, specifically only for the evaluation of SCC arising in the oropharynx. Numerous methodologies exist for direct testing for HPV; however, in situ hybridization is the most universally used method allowing for screening of all known high-risk HPV types (16, 18, 31, 33, 35, 39, 45, 51, 52, 56, 58, and 66) in one test on standard paraffin tissue sections.[66,67]

Limited availability of this methodology for testing in the community and concern for lower sensitivity compared with polymerase chain reaction (PCR) led to the evaluation of p16 as a surrogate marker for the presence of HPV in tumor cells. The tumor suppressor gene p16 is involved in cell cycle regulation that shows diffuse overexpression (cytoplasmic and nuclear) in tumor cells infected by HPV using standard immunohistochemical techniques. The mechanism of p16 overexpression is theorized to be secondary to viral components (E6 and E7) interfering with the function of Rb and p53 leading to compensatory upregulation of p16. Early analysis of clinical trial tumor samples showed p16 expression in primary OPSCC tissue strongly correlated with HPV status and improved survival.[13] Although the association between p16 expression and HPV+ is strong in the oropharynx, p16 expression in other HNSCC tissue sites may be unrelated to HPV (as confirmed by negative PCR validation in multiple studies) stressing the need to perform a concurrent direct test for HPV confirmation if testing tissue outside of the oropharynx. Currently, HPV tumor status is only used as a prognostic and etiologic factor; however, ongoing clinical trials are looking at treatment modifications for HPV+ tumors to reduce the long-term morbidities in this younger cancer population. Additionally, although clinical trials specific to OPSCC prevention through HPV vaccination are infeasible, the implementation of the HPV vaccination in the population holds the potential for reducing the overall incidence of HPV. Vaccination is theorized to ultimately result in reducing HPV-associated SCC in the head and neck in the coming decades as HPVs in the oropharynx are the same high-risk types that cause cervical cancer and that the spread of HPV to the oropharynx has been linked to changes in sexual practices and increased sexual partners.

MOLECULAR ALTERATIONS IN HNSCC
Tp53 and EGFR

Many HNSCCs overexpress the EGFR a gene involved in cell proliferation, angiogenesis, migration, adhesion, and invasion. This observation led to clinical trials and ultimately Food and Drug Administration approval of cetuximab, a monoclonal antibody directed against EGFR, as an adjuvant treatment with radiation in HNSCC. However, no biomarkers have been identified to date with regard to response or resistance to EGFR inhibitors in HNSCC.

Mutation of the TP53 tumor suppressor gene is the most common and earliest genetic alteration associated with HNSCC.[68] Missense mutations involving the DNA-binding domain of TP53 gene are seen in more than 50% of all conventional/tobacco-related HNSCC. Testing for the TP53 mutation in biopsies of HNSCC and its precursors is labor intensive and not feasible in a clinical laboratory. Moreover, currently there are no specific treatment guidelines for HNSCC with TP53 mutations. With the development of next-generation sequencing and array technologies allowing for sequencing/screening of whole genes with minimal tumor tissue, new areas of research are ongoing, exploring TP53's association with outcomes and therapies. This research may lead to new, personalized care for patients with HNSCC.[69]

ACKNOWLEDGMENTS

The authors thank Ms. Rhonda Whitmeyer, University of Texas School of Dentistry at Houston, for editorial support.

REFERENCES

1. Parkin DM, Bray F, Ferlay J, et al. Global cancer statistics, 2002. CA Cancer J Clin 2005;55(2):74–108.
2. Warnakulasuriya S. Global epidemiology of oral and oropharyngeal cancer. Oral Oncol 2009; 45(4–5):309–16.
3. Siegel R, Naishadham D, Jemal A. Cancer statistics, 2013. CA Cancer J Clin 2013;63(1):11–30.
4. Sturgis EM, Cinciripini PM. Trends in head and neck cancer incidence in relation to smoking prevalence: an emerging epidemic of human papillomavirus-associated cancers? Cancer 2007; 110(7):1429–35.
5. Ramqvist T, Dalianis T. Oropharyngeal cancer epidemic and human papillomavirus. Emerg Infect Dis 2010;16(11):1671–7.
6. Carvalho AL, Nishimoto IN, Califano JA, et al. Trends in incidence and prognosis for head and neck cancer in the United States: a site-specific analysis of the SEER database. Int J Cancer 2005;114(5):806–16.
7. Fakhry C, D'Souza G. Discussing the diagnosis of HPV-OSCC: common questions and answers. Oral Oncol 2013;49(9):863–71.
8. Blot WJ, McLaughlin JK, Winn DM, et al. Smoking and drinking in relation to oral and pharyngeal cancer. Cancer Res 1988;48(11):3282–7.
9. Travasso C. Betel quid chewing is responsible for half of oral cancer cases in India, finds study. BMJ 2013;347:f7536.
10. Rodu B, Jansson C. Smokeless tobacco and oral cancer: a review of the risks and determinants. Crit Rev Oral Biol Med 2004;15(5):252–63.
11. Petti S, Masood M, Messano GA, et al. Alcohol is not a risk factor for oral cancer in nonsmoking, betel quid non-chewing individuals. A meta-analysis update. Ann Ig 2013;25(1):3–14.
12. Kreimer AR, Clifford GM, Boyle P, et al. Human papillomavirus types in head and neck squamous cell carcinomas worldwide: a systematic review. Cancer Epidemiol Biomarkers Prev 2005;14(2): 467–75.
13. Ang KK, Harris J, Wheeler R, et al. Human papillomavirus and survival of patients with oropharyngeal cancer. N Engl J Med 2010;363(1):24–35.
14. Levitus M, Joenje H, de Winter JP. The Fanconi anemia pathway of genomic maintenance. Cell Oncol 2006;28(1–2):3–29.
15. Kutler DI, Auerbach AD, Satagopan J, et al. High incidence of head and neck squamous cell

carcinoma in patients with Fanconi anemia. Arch Otolaryngol Head Neck Surg 2003;129(1):106–12.

16. Masserot C, Peffault de Latour R, Rocha V, et al. Head and neck squamous cell carcinoma in 13 patients with Fanconi anemia after hematopoietic stem cell transplantation. Cancer 2008;113(12):3315–22.

17. Bessler M, Wilson DB, Mason PJ. Dyskeratosis congenita. FEBS Lett 2010;584(17):3831–8.

18. Scheckenbach K, Wagenmann M, Freund M, et al. Squamous cell carcinomas of the head and neck in Fanconi anemia: risk, prevention, therapy, and the need for guidelines. Klin Padiatr 2012;224(3):132–8.

19. Vigneswaran N, Tilashalski K, Rodu B, et al. Tobacco use and cancer. A reappraisal. Oral Surg Oral Med Oral Pathol Oral Radiol Endod 1995; 80(2):178–82.

20. Centers for Disease Control and Prevention (CDC). Human papillomavirus-associated cancers - United States, 2004-2008. MMWR Morb Mortal Wkly Rep 2012;61:258–61.

21. Chen AY, Myers JN. Cancer of the oral cavity. Dis Mon 2001;47(7):275–361.

22. Ridge JA, Glisson BS, Lango MN, et al. Head and neck tumors. In: Haller DE, Wagman LD, Camphausen KA, et al, editors. Cancer management: a multidisciplinary approach, medical, surgical & radiation oncology. 14th edition. Norwalk, CT: UBM Medica; 2011. p. 1–42.

23. Patel SC, Carpenter WR, Tyree S, et al. Increasing incidence of oral tongue squamous cell carcinoma in young white women, age 18 to 44 years. J Clin Oncol 2011;29(11):1488–94.

24. Schantz SP, Yu GP. Head and neck cancer incidence trends in young Americans, 1973-1997, with a special analysis for tongue cancer. Arch Otolaryngol Head Neck Surg 2002;128(3): 268–74.

25. Shiboski CH, Schmidt BL, Jordan RC. Tongue and tonsil carcinoma: increasing trends in the U.S. population ages 20-44 years. Cancer 2005;103(9): 1843–9.

26. Harris SL, Kimple RJ, Hayes DN, et al. Never-smokers, never-drinkers: unique clinical subgroup of young patients with head and neck squamous cell cancers. Head Neck 2010;32(4):499–503.

27. Vargas H, Pitman KT, Johnson JT, et al. More aggressive behavior of squamous cell carcinoma of the anterior tongue in young women. Laryngoscope 2000;110(10 Pt 1):1623–6.

28. Sano D, Myers JN. Metastasis of squamous cell carcinoma of the oral tongue. Cancer Metastasis Rev 2007;26(3–4):645–62.

29. Warnakulasuriya S, Johnson NW, van der Waal I. Nomenclature and classification of potentially malignant disorders of the oral mucosa. J Oral Pathol Med 2007;36(10):575–80.

30. Caporaso NE. Why precursors matter. Cancer Epidemiol Biomarkers Prev 2013;22(4):518–20.

31. Napier SS, Speight PM. Natural history of potentially malignant oral lesions and conditions: an overview of the literature. J Oral Pathol Med 2008; 37(1):1–10.

32. Gillenwater AM, Vigneswaran N, Fatani H, et al. Proliferative verrucous leukoplakia (PVL): recognition and differentiation from conventional leukoplakia and mimics! Head Neck 2013. [Epub ahead of print].

33. Gillenwater AM, Vigneswaran N, Fatani H, et al. Proliferative verrucous leukoplakia (PVL): a review of an elusive pathologic entity! Adv Anat Pathol 2013;20(6):416–23.

34. Zain RB, Ikeda N, Gupta PC, et al. Oral mucosal lesions associated with betel quid, areca nut and tobacco chewing habits: consensus from a workshop held in Kuala Lumpur, Malaysia, November 25-27, 1996. J Oral Pathol Med 1999; 28(1):1–4.

35. Eisen D. The clinical features, malignant potential, and systemic associations of oral lichen planus: a study of 723 patients. J Am Acad Dermatol 2002; 46(2):207–14.

36. Lovas JG, Harsanyi BB, ElGeneidy AK. Oral lichenoid dysplasia: a clinicopathologic analysis. Oral Surg Oral Med Oral Pathol 1989;68(1):57–63.

37. Zhang L, Cheng X, Li Y, et al. High frequency of allelic loss in dysplastic lichenoid lesions. Lab Invest 2000;80(2):233–7.

38. Epstein JB, Guneri P, Boyacioglu H, et al. The limitations of the clinical oral examination in detecting dysplastic oral lesions and oral squamous cell carcinoma. J Am Dent Assoc 2012;143(12): 1332–42.

39. Shin D, Vigneswaran N, Gillenwater A, et al. Advances in fluorescence imaging techniques to detect oral cancer and its precursors. Future Oncol 2010;6(7):1143–54.

40. Lingen MW, Kalmar JR, Karrison T, et al. Critical evaluation of diagnostic aids for the detection of oral cancer. Oral Oncol 2008;44(1):10–22.

41. Speight PM. Update on oral epithelial dysplasia and progression to cancer. Head Neck Pathol 2007;1(1):61–6.

42. Mithani SK, Mydlarz WK, Grumbine FL, et al. Molecular genetics of premalignant oral lesions. Oral Dis 2007;13(2):126–33.

43. Zhang L, Poh CF, Williams M, et al. Loss of heterozygosity (LOH) profiles–validated risk predictors for progression to oral cancer. Cancer Prev Res (Phila) 2012;5(9):1081–9.

44. Brennan M, Migliorati CA, Lockhart PB, et al. Management of oral epithelial dysplasia: a review. Oral Surg Oral Med Oral Pathol Oral Radiol Endod 2007;103(Suppl):S19.e11–2.

45. Arnaoutakis D, Bishop J, Westra W, et al. Recurrence patterns and management of oral cavity premalignant lesions. Oral Oncol 2013;49(8): 814–7.

46. Mehanna HM, Rattay T, Smith J, et al. Treatment and follow-up of oral dysplasia - a systematic review and meta-analysis. Head Neck 2009;31(12): 1600–9.

47. Meltzer C. Surgical management of oral and mucosal dysplasias: the case for laser excision. J Oral Maxillofac Surg 2007;65(2):293–5.

48. Saito T, Sugiura C, Hirai A, et al. Development of squamous cell carcinoma from pre-existent oral leukoplakia: with respect to treatment modality. Int J Oral Maxillofac Surg 2001;30(1): 49–53.

49. Wong SJ, Campbell B, Massey B, et al. A phase I trial of aminolevulinic acid-photodynamic therapy for treatment of oral leukoplakia. Oral Oncol 2013; 49(9):970–6.

50. Saba N, Hurwitz SJ, Kono S, et al. Chemoprevention of head and neck cancer with celecoxib and erlotinib: results of a phase 1b and pharmacokinetic study. Cancer Prev Res 2014;7(3):283–91.

51. El-Mofty SK, Patil S. Human papillomavirus (HPV)-related oropharyngeal nonkeratinizing squamous cell carcinoma: characterization of a distinct phenotype. Oral Surg Oral Med Oral Pathol Oral Radiol Endod 2006;101(3):339–45.

52. Savagner P. The epithelial-mesenchymal transition (EMT) phenomenon. Ann Oncol 2010;21(Suppl 7): vii89–92.

53. Tai SK, Li WY, Chu PY, et al. Risks and clinical implications of perineural invasion in T1-2 oral tongue squamous cell carcinoma. Head Neck 2012;34(7): 994–1001.

54. Yuen AP, Ho CM, Chow TL, et al. Prospective randomized study of selective neck dissection versus observation for N0 neck of early tongue carcinoma. Head Neck 2009;31(6):765–72.

55. Sparano A, Weinstein G, Chalian A, et al. Multivariate predictors of occult neck metastasis in early oral tongue cancer. Otolaryngol Head Neck Surg 2004;131(4):472–6.

56. Zhang T, Lubek JE, Salama A, et al. Treatment of cT1N0M0 tongue cancer: outcome and prognostic parameters. J Oral Maxillofac Surg 2014;72(2): 406–14.

57. Mohit-Tabatabai MA, Sobel HJ, Rush BF, et al. Relation of thickness of floor of mouth stage I and II cancers to regional metastasis. Am J Surg 1986;152(4):351–3.

58. Chandler K, Vance C, Budnick S, et al. Muscle invasion in oral tongue squamous cell carcinoma as a predictor of nodal status and local recurrence: just as effective as depth of invasion? Head Neck Pathol 2011;5(4):359–63.

59. Brandwein-Gensler M, Teixeira MS, Lewis CM, et al. Oral squamous cell carcinoma: histologic risk assessment, but not margin status, is strongly predictive of local disease-free and overall survival. Am J Surg Pathol 2005;29(2):167–78.

60. Hinni ML, Ferlito A, Brandwein-Gensler MS, et al. Surgical margins in head and neck cancer: a contemporary review. Head Neck 2013;35(9):1362–70.

61. Slootweg PJ, Hordijk GJ, Schade Y, et al. Treatment failure and margin status in head and neck cancer. A critical view on the potential value of molecular pathology. Oral Oncol 2002;38(5):500–3.

62. Johnson JT, Myers EN, Bedetti CD, et al. Cervical lymph node metastases. Incidence and implications of extracapsular carcinoma. Arch Otolaryngol 1985;111(8):534–7.

63. Myers JN, Greenberg JS, Mo V, et al. Extracapsular spread. A significant predictor of treatment failure in patients with squamous cell carcinoma of the tongue. Cancer 2001;92(12):3030–6.

64. Gruber G, Bonetti M, Nasi ML, et al. Prognostic value of extracapsular tumor spread for locoregional control in premenopausal patients with node-positive breast cancer treated with classical cyclophosphamide, methotrexate, and fluorouracil: long-term observations from International Breast Cancer Study Group Trial VI. J Clin Oncol 2005; 23(28):7089–97.

65. Edge SB, Byrd DR, Compton CC, et al, editors. AJCC cancer staging manual. 7th edition. New York: Springer; 2009.

66. Schache AG, Liloglou T, Risk JM, et al. Evaluation of human papilloma virus diagnostic testing in oropharyngeal squamous cell carcinoma: sensitivity, specificity, and prognostic discrimination. Clin Cancer Res 2011;17(19):6262–71.

67. Duray A, Descamps G, Arafa M, et al. High incidence of high-risk HPV in benign and malignant lesions of the larynx. Int J Oncol 2011;39(1):51–9.

68. Rothenberg SM, Ellisen LW. The molecular pathogenesis of head and neck squamous cell carcinoma. J Clin Invest 2012;122(6):1951–7.

69. Skinner HD, Sandulache VC, Ow TJ, et al. TP53 disruptive mutations lead to head and neck cancer treatment failure through inhibition of radiation-induced senescence. Clin Cancer Res 2012; 18(1):290–300.

Use of Porous Space Maintainers in Staged Mandibular Reconstruction

Allan M. Henslee, PhD[a], Patrick P. Spicer, PhD[a],
Sarita R. Shah, BS[a], Alexander M. Tatara, BS[a],
F. Kurtis Kasper, PhD[a], Antonios G. Mikos, PhD[a],
Mark E. Wong, DDS[b],*

KEYWORDS

- Mandibular reconstruction • Polymethylmethacrylate space maintainer • Implant fabrication

KEY POINTS

- The success of mandibular reconstructions depends not only on restoring the form and function of lost bone but also on the preservation of the overlying soft tissue layer.
- In this case study, 5 porous polymethylmethacrylate space maintainers fabricated via patient-specific molds were implanted initially to maintain the vitality of the overlying oral mucosa during staged mandibular reconstructions. Three of the 5 patients healed well, whereas the other 2 patients developed dehiscences, most likely due to a thin layer of soft tissue overlying the implant.
- The results presented provide evidence that a larger investigation of space maintainers fabricated using this method is warranted.

INTRODUCTION

Continuity defects of the mandible can be the result of tumor resection or trauma. In cases involving high-velocity projectiles, blast injuries, or locally aggressive tumors, bone loss is often associated with loss or compromise of the overlying soft tissue.[1,2] The goals of reconstruction must therefore include not only strategies for the replacement of bone but also methods to restore or preserve the overlying soft tissue.

CLINICAL CHALLENGE

Several techniques are available for the reconstruction of osseous defects of the mandible, with the gold standard remaining autologous bone transplantation.[3,4] When nonvascularized bone grafts are used, definitive reconstruction is often delayed until a clean wound environment without oral communication is present.[5] Without this delay to allow the soft tissue envelope to heal, an increased incidence of wound dehiscence and graft infection has been reported.[6,7] During healing of the oral tissues, the soft tissue adjacent to the bony defect prolapses into the area filling the space between the bony segments. When secondary reconstruction is attempted several months later, this tissue must be dissected or excised to re-create the defect to be filled with bone. Nerves, nerve grafts, and blood vessels contained within this interspersed soft tissue may be injured during dissection. The concept of space maintenance was developed to assist these staged reconstructive procedures by preserving the soft tissue envelope surrounding the bone defect, creating a pocket for the insertion of a bone graft.

Space maintenance involves the temporary implantation of an alloplastic material into a defect

[a] Department of Bioengineering, Rice University, 6500 Main Street, Houston, TX 77005, USA; [b] Department of Oral of Maxillofacial Surgery, University of Texas Health Science Center, 7500 Cambridge Street, Houston, TX 77054, USA
* Corresponding author.
E-mail address: mark.e.wong@uth.tmc.edu

Oral Maxillofacial Surg Clin N Am 26 (2014) 143–149
http://dx.doi.org/10.1016/j.coms.2014.01.002
1042-3699/14/$ – see front matter © 2014 Elsevier Inc. All rights reserved.

to prevent wound contracture into the space normally occupied by bone.[5] Currently, the most widely used alloplastic material for craniofacial reconstruction is polymethylmethacrylate (PMMA) bone cement, an acrylic-based resin.[8] PMMA has also been used in skeletal space maintenance applications[5,6,9] and specifically within the craniofacial complex.[10] PMMA is strong, nondegradable, easily moldable, inert, and simple to mix intraoperatively, making it an ideal material for temporary placement into irregularly shaped defects.[5] Unfortunately, complications such as wound dehiscence and implant exposure are not infrequent and result from compromised soft tissue healing over an implant.[5–7] Once an implant is exposed in the oral cavity, secondary contamination with saliva and oral organisms occurs very quickly, and inflammation, infection, and secondary fibrosis can compromise the wound bed if the implants are not removed immediately.

In addition, intraoperative formation of PMMA space maintainers has been associated with local thermal or chemical necrosis as a result of high curing temperatures and leaching of residual monomer (methylmethacrylate, MMA).[11,12] These concerns are addressed with several innovations and the authors' early experiences with optimized spacer technology are presented.

TECHNICAL INNOVATIONS

Recent innovations in craniofacial surgery as well as research into biomaterial-tissue interfaces have identified several technologies capable of improving the performance and biocompatibility of space maintainers. First, advances in computer-aided modeling techniques allow the development of accurate and affordable surgical models.[13–15] From these models, an anatomically correct template can be fabricated for a space maintainer to fit the proposed defect accurately before surgery. In addition, investigations into material surfaces properties have focused on the creation of porosity within implants to improve retention and soft tissue integration.[16–18] A porous structure allows fibrovascular tissue ingrowth, which improves wound healing and the formation of a stable interface. In the work described here, low porosity was introduced into PMMA implants to facilitate the attachment of the overlying soft tissue layer through mechanical interlocking while minimizing hard and soft tissue ingrowth. Combining this technique with computer-aided modeling allowed for the fabrication of porous PMMA implants customized to fit into a bony resection defect produced during the treatment of benign mandibular pathologic abnormality.

Fabrication of space maintainers preoperatively using molds produced from patient-specific 3-dimensional (3D) models provides several advantages over in situ fabricated implants. The device dimensions approximate the defect dimensions very closely, reducing the time it takes to mix, mold, and trim implants produced intraoperatively. Also, by fabricating a spacer ex vivo, problems associated with intraoperative molding of PMMA such as local tissue damage injury through thermal or chemical injury can be avoided. The polymerization of PMMA is highly exothermic and temperatures reaching 110°C on polymerization have been reported.[19] By fabricating implants outside the surgical defect, tissue necrosis associated with temperature rise is eliminated. Second, MMA monomer released from PMMA during polymerization is toxic to cells, but previous studies have found that toxicity is reduced to negligible levels after 48 hours of polymerization with solid PMMA samples.[11,20] Studies on the actual formulation of porous PMMA used in patients (30 wt% carboxymethylcellulose [CMC]) demonstrated minimal release of MMA after 3 days.[21]

One potential problem of using prefabricated implants relates to the ability to predict surgical margins accurately on 3D models. Although radiographic data are usually accurate, final margins are not confirmed until surgery. In view of this, it has been found prudent to fashion larger spacers that can be trimmed after the resection has been completed.

ADVANTAGES OF POROUS SPACE MAINTAINERS

The use of porous PMMA in this study has many advantages over conventional solid PMMA space maintainers. Past clinical studies have shown that porosity can play an important role in implant attachment to the surrounding soft tissue[11,17,18,22] because the pores of a space maintainer provide "anchorage points" for healing tissue to infiltrate, thereby achieving mechanical attachment over the entire surface of a flap and not just at the incision margins where sutures are placed. This enhanced mechanical support for the flap is thought to reduce the incidence of dehiscence. This hypothesis was tested by in vivo studies demonstrating that porous space maintainers were associated with fewer dehiscences compared with nonporous space maintainers when implanted in segmental rabbit mandibular defects.[23,24] In one study, it was postulated that porous PMMA samples with reduced porosity (30 vs 40 wt%) performed better because they had less of an inflammatory response. Implants fabricated in the current study were designed and confirmed to contain porosity values similar to that of porous space maintainers optimized from this previous in vivo study (30 wt% CMC).[23] Overall, the fabrication method used to create porous PMMA in this study was reliable and effective.

IMPLANT FABRICATION

Computed tomographic scans were used to create 3D starch models of each patient's mandible (**Fig. 1**A). Each model was then mounted on a plaster of Paris base, which registered the inferior border of the mandible (see **Fig. 1**B) and provided a reference for realigning the mandibular anatomy after it had been sectioned to duplicate the planned surgical procedure. The section containing the pathologic abnormality was removed from the model and a wax spacer template was molded to match the dimensions of the defect (see **Fig. 1**C, D). Use of a plaster of Paris base plate preserves the original dimensions of the mandible while molding the spacer template. In addition to molding a template, the 3D models were also used to bend a reconstruction bone plate before surgery to reduce operative time (see **Fig. 1**B, D). To produce a mold for the actual PMMA spacer, an elastomeric silicone polymer was conformed around the wax template. Once the silicone set, it was cut in half to create a negative mold of the proposed space maintainer (see **Fig. 1**E). Porous PMMA fabricated by mixing clinically available high-viscosity bone cement with 30 wt% carboxymethylcellulose (9 wt% in dH_2O) was then placed into the molds to produce the final space maintenance device (see **Fig. 1**F).

CASE SERIES

A series of 5 patients were treated for benign mandibular pathologic abnormality at the authors' institution. Following resection of the affected portion of the mandible, a porous PMMA spacer was placed into the defect and secured in position with a reconstructed bone plate and multiple locking positional bone screws. The series comprised 3 patients with a diagnosis of ameloblastoma, one case of a keratocystic odontogenic tumor, and one case of a glandular odontogenic cyst. Before implantation of the preformed spacers, the devices were soaked in bacitracin solution to mitigate against the risk of bacterial contamination. The space maintainers were trimmed to fit the exact dimensions of the defect at the time of surgery with either a reciprocating saw or an acrylic reduction burr. In addition, the surface of

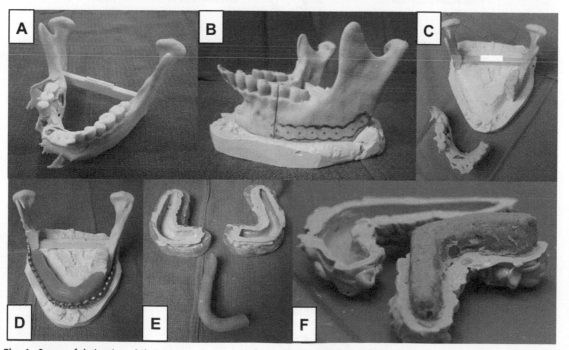

Fig. 1. Spacer fabrication. (*A*) A 3D starch model of a mandible produced from computed tomographic data and 3D printing. (*B*) A mandibular model and a plaster of Paris base plate. An outline of the proposed location of the reconstruction bone plate is visible along the inferior border of the mandible. (*C*) The model is shown with the resected section removed. (*D*) A hand-molded wax spacer occupying the proposed defect. (*E*) The wax spacer shown next to its negative mold fabricated from silicone. (*F*) A porous PMMA space maintainer (untrimmed) shown within the silicone mold.

space maintainers was smoothed to remove sharp edges or irregularities from the fabrication process to prevent perforation of the overlying soft tissue flaps. A summary of the 5 cases is presented in **Fig. 2**.

CLINICAL OUTCOMES

Although generally positive, the porous PMMA space maintainers did not avoid wound dehiscences in all cases as was originally hoped. Two of the 5 patients experienced implant exposure and the subsequent inflammatory response required removal of these devices prematurely. In the remaining 3 cases, all implants were retained satisfactorily and 2 of the 3 patients have undergone subsequent bone grafting with excellent functional and esthetic results (**Fig. 3**).

The 2 patients that required removal of the spacers exhibited both qualitative and quantitative deficiencies in soft tissue overlying the mandibular defects and required additional adjunctive measures to support successful bone grafting. In one case a pedicled buccinator myomucosal flap was rotated into the defect before a successful bone graft was performed. In the second case, where the defect extended from the left mandibular body to the right mandibular angle, a vascularized free fibula transfer was performed with a skin pedicle.

Retrospective analysis of these failures suggested several factors that could have contributed to implant exposure. In one case, a large porous spacer extending across the mandibular symphysis became exposed in the midline following breakdown of the incision (**Fig. 4**). In a previous study analyzing mandibular implants, van Gemert and colleagues[4] found that implants reconstructing the anterior mandible were significantly more likely to fail. It has been hypothesized that devices

Patient (age/sex)	Tumor/Defect Description	Space Maintainer/Tumor	Space Maintainer Result	Final Result
1 (28/M)	• Ameloblastoma • 10cm segmental defect across the midline • Significant soft tissue removal		• Dehiscence observed 12 days postoperatively across midline of SM	• Reconstructed with a free fibula flap and skin paddle
2 (48/M)	• Keratocystic odontogenic tumor • 12cm defect including the angle and condyle		• SM healed without complication and remained for 15 months • No observed dehiscence	• Reconstructed with block and particulate bone graft
3 (41/M)	• Glandular odontongenic cyst • 6.5cm segmental defect		• SM healed with complication and remained for 4 months • No observed dehiscence	• Reconstructed with block and particulate bone graft
4 (69/M)	• Ameloblastoma • 4cm segmental defect • Significant soft tissue removal		• Dehiscence observed 6 weeks postoperatively with a 2cm exposure on the lateral aspect of SM	• Reconstructed with block and particulate bone graft
5 (20/M)	• Ameloblastoma • 7cm segmental defect		• SM healed without complication and complete soft tissue coverage was observed 2 months postoperatively	• Awaiting reconstruction

Fig. 2. Summary of case series. SM, space maintainer.

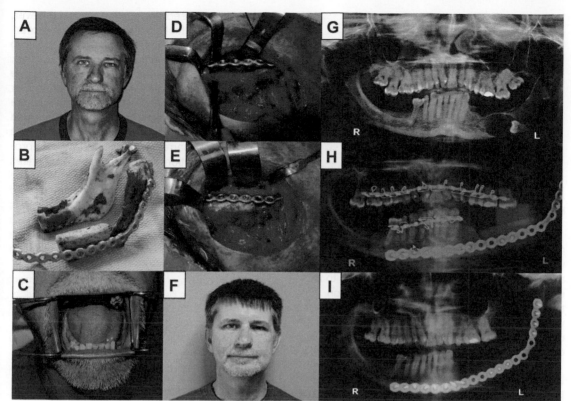

Fig. 3. Pictures from case 2. (*A*) Patient before surgery. (*B*) Section of removed bone shown next to space maintainer along with rib graft. (*C*) Twelve weeks postoperatively showing healed mucosa over the space maintainer. (*D*) Space maintainer just before removal showing vascularized tissue envelope. (*E*) Reconstruction performed with block and particulate bone graft. (*F*) Patient following reconstruction. (*G*) Radiograph taken before surgery. (*H*) Radiograph following initial excision surgery. (*I*) Radiograph following final reconstruction.

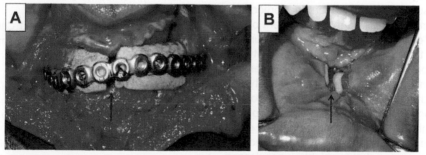

Fig. 4. (*A*) Implantation of spacer extending across the mandibular symphysis (*arrow*), and (*B*) subsequent exposure of the implant across the symphysis (*arrow*) 12 days postoperatively.

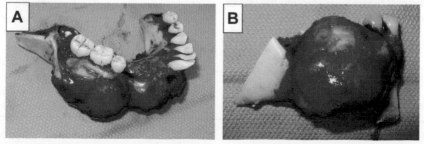

Fig. 5. Bony resections including the removal of large sections of overlying soft tissue. (*A*) Case 1; (*B*) case 4.

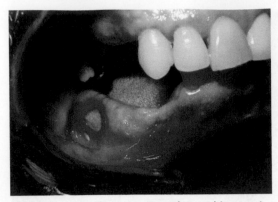

Fig. 6. Lateral implant exposure observed in case 4.

or grafts in the anterior portion of the mandible were subject to greater flexion forces and these adverse mechanical conditions could lead to incision failure. Another important observation was that implant exposure occurred in patients in whom bony resection included the removal of overlying soft tissue (**Fig. 5**), leading to a thin flap over the implant.

The significance of flap thickness was illustrated well with one case of implant exposure through the lateral aspect of the oral closure and not along the incision line (**Fig. 6**). A reduced thickness of soft tissue can also increase the tension applied to sutures, and when this is the case, soft tissue flaps or grafts may be required to decrease the likelihood of implant exposure.[25]

Contributing to the definitive reconstruction of osseous tissues, the regeneration and remodeling of newly formed bone is highly dependent on the migration of cells into the defect from surrounding tissues, and this relies heavily on the cellularity and vascularity of the recipient site.[26,27] With respect to the current study, the degree of cellularity and vascularity of the recipient site is directly related to the amount and health of the overlying soft tissue. Although difficult to quantify clinically, gross observations of the recipient sites during secondary operations revealed a highly vascularized envelope of soft tissue into which the graft was placed. By improving the vascularity and thickness of the overlying soft tissue layer through the use of porous space maintainers in conjunction with soft tissue flaps, the likelihood of success for subsequent tissue grafts/flaps is increased.

SUMMARY

Porous PMMA space maintainers fabricated preoperatively from patient-specific 3D models assist in the staged reconstruction of mandibular defects by decreasing operative time and improving the fidelity of the osseous reconstruction. However, the amount and thickness of the soft tissue overlying the spacer are important considerations in case selection. When tissue is missing or thinned, adjunctive procedures to augment the soft tissue coverage of the spacer must be performed or erosion through the flap with implant exposure may occur. Exposed spacers are poorly tolerated and secondary infection and soft tissue fibrosis can lead to a scarred wound bed and compromised reconstruction. Although the series of cases was relatively small, the results presented here provide evidence that a larger investigation of space maintainers fabricated in this method is warranted. The use of porous space maintainers in mandibular reconstructions is a viable technique that holds the potential to benefit both patients and clinicians alike.

REFERENCES

1. Rodriguez E, Martin M, Bluebond-Langner R, et al. Multiplanar distraction osteogenesis of fibula free flaps used for secondary reconstruction of traumatic maxillary defects. J Craniofac Surg 2006; 17(5):883–8.

2. Posnick JC, Wells M, Zuker R. Use of the free fibular flap in the immediate reconstruction of pediatric mandibular tumors: report of cases. J Oral Maxillofac Surg 1993;51(2):189–96.

3. Gadre P, Ramanojam S, Patankar A, et al. Nonvascularized bone grafting for mandibular reconstruction: myth or reality? J Craniofac Surg 2011;22(5): 1727–35.

4. van Gemert JT, van Es RJ, Van Cann EM, et al. Nonvascularized bone grafts for segmental reconstruction of the mandible–a reappraisal. J Oral Maxillofac Surg 2009;67(7):1446–52.

5. Goodger NM, Wang J, Smagalski GW, et al. Methylmethacrylate as a space maintainer in mandibular reconstruction. J Oral Maxillofac Surg 2005;63(7): 1048–51.

6. Govila A. Use of methyl methacrylate in bone reconstruction. Br J Plast Surg 1990;43(2):210–6.

7. Benoist M. Experience with 220 cases of mandibular reconstruction. J Maxillofac Surg 1978;6(1):40–9.

8. Filho RC, Oliveira TM, Neto NL, et al. Reconstruction of bony facial contour deficiencies with polymethylmethacrylate implants: case report. J Appl Oral Sci 2011;19(4):426–30.

9. Wright S, Bekiroglu F, Whear NM, et al. Use of Palacos R-40 with gentamicin to reconstruct temporal defects after maxillofacial reconstructions with temporalis flaps. Br J Oral Maxillofac Surg 2006;44(6): 531–3.

10. Spetzger U, Vougioukas V, Schipper J. Materials and techniques for osseous skull reconstruction.

Minim Invasive Ther Allied Technol 2010;19(2): 110–21.

11. Lu JX, Huang ZW, Tropiano P. Human biological reactions at the interface between bone tissue and polymethylmethacrylate cement. J Mater Sci Mater Med 2002;13(8):803–9.

12. O'Dowd-Booth C, White J, Smitham P, et al. Bone cement: perioperative issues, orthopaedic applications and future developments. J Perioper Pract 2011;21(9):304–8.

13. Hannen EJ. Recreating the original contour in tumor deformed mandibles for plate adapting. Int J Oral Maxillofac Surg 2006;35(2):183–5.

14. Cheng HT, Wu CI, Tseng CS, et al. The occlusion-adjusted prefabricated 3D mirror image templates by computer simulation: the image-guided navigation system application in difficult cases of head and neck reconstruction. Ann Plast Surg 2009;63(5):517–21. http://dx.doi.org/10.1097/SAP. 0b013e31819349b9.

15. Fernandes R, DiPasquale J. Computer-aided surgery using 3D rendering of maxillofacial pathology and trauma. Int J Med Robot 2007;3(3):203–6.

16. Liu J, Gottfried O, Cole C, et al. Porous polyethylene implant for cranioplasty and skull base reconstruction. Neurosurg Focus 2004;16(3):ECP1.

17. Bruens ML, Pieterman H, de Wijn JR, et al. Porous polymethylmethacrylate as bone substitute in the craniofacial area. J Craniofac Surg 2003;14(1):63–8.

18. van Mullem P, Vaandrager JM, Nicolai J, et al. Implantation of porous acrylic cement in soft tissues: an animal and human biopsy histological study. Biomaterials 1990;11(5):299–304.

19. Meyer P, Lautenschlager E, Moore B. On the setting properties of acrylic bone cement. J Bone Joint Surg Am 1973;55(1):149–56.

20. Granchi D, Stea S, Ciapetti G, et al. In vitro effects of bone cements on the cell cycle of osteoblast-like cells. Biomaterials 1995;16(15):1187–92.

21. Wang L, Yoon DM, Spicer PP, et al. Characterization of porous polymethylmethacrylate space maintainers for craniofacial reconstruction. J Biomed Mater Res B Appl Biomater 2013;101B(5):813–25.

22. Van Mullem P, De Wijn JR, Vaandrager JM. Porous acrylic cement: evaluation of a novel implant material. Ann Plast Surg 1988;21(6):576–82.

23. Kretlow JD, Shi M, Young S, et al. Evaluation of soft tissue coverage over porous polymethylmethacrylate space maintainers within nonhealing alveolar bone defects. Tissue Eng Part C Methods 2010; 16(6):1427–38.

24. Nguyen C, Young S, Kretlow JD, et al. Surface characteristics of biomaterials used for space maintenance in a mandibular defect: a pilot animal study. J Oral Maxillofac Surg 2010;69(1):11–8.

25. Palacci P, Nowzari H. Soft tissue enhancement around dental implants. Periodontol 2000 2008;47: 113–32.

26. Pogrel MA, Podlesh S, Anthony JP, et al. A comparison of vascularized and nonvascularized bone grafts for reconstruction of mandibular continuity defects. J Oral Maxillofac Surg 1997;55(11): 1200–6.

27. Marx R. Clinical application of bone biology to mandibular and maxillary reconstruction. Clin Plast Surg 1994;21(3):377–92.

Pitfalls in Determining Head and Neck Surgical Margins

Y. Etan Weinstock, MD[a],*, Ibrahim Alava III, MD[a],
Eric J. Dierks, DMD, MD[b]

KEYWORDS

• Oral cavity • Cancer • Resection • Frozen • Margin • Shrinkage • Autofluorescent
• Hypermethylation

KEY POINTS

• Adequate extirpation of solid tumors of the head and neck require clear margins for increased survival.
• Oral cavity cancers remain, for the most part, surgical diseases that require a thorough understanding of anatomy, lymphatic drainage, and surgical oncologic technique.
• Current margin assessment planning necessitates preoperative planning, intraoperative evaluation, and a close relationship with pathology.
• Newer techniques are being developed to detect positive margins on the molecular level as well as detect dysplastic changes much quicker in the surveillance phase.

INTRODUCTION

In the twenty-first century, much like in the nineteenth and twentieth centuries, the inadequate removal of tumor from the primary site remains the overwhelming cause of failure and death of patients with head and neck squamous cell carcinoma (HNSCC).[1] Oncologic surgeons have long adhered to the Halsteadean principle of strict en bloc resection of all cancerous tissue, including an adequate margin of normal-appearing tissue to encompass all vestiges of microscopic, local tumor extension. However, the extent of normal-appearing tissue that requires surgical resection remains unclear. There are various factors that may lead to difficult margin assessments and also divergent opinions of what constitutes a "close" or worrisome margin. Additionally, there are multiple anatomic and histologic factors that may affect oncologic outcomes regardless of extent of resection. In the current era of evolving

minimally invasive endoscopic surgical approaches and increased emphasis on molecular medicine, classical surgical margins may be unachievable and perhaps even archaic. Last, phenotypic expression of malignancy occurs only after the genetic malformation has occurred. In this review, we intend to evaluate the current opinion in margin assessment, illustrate potential shortcomings in these assessments, and postulate on ways that margin studies and tumor biology may become instructive in dictating surgical approaches.

HISTORICAL PERSPECTIVE

The traditional definition of an oncologic surgical margin is an anatomic clearance of all neoplastic tissue in a 3-dimensional orientation. Thus, it is implied that all cancerous cells are encompassed within the resection specimen. However, despite this assertion, local tumor recurrence can still

[a] Department of Otorhinolaryngology, University of Texas Health Science Center at Houston, 6431 Fannin Street MSB 5.031, Houston TX 77030, USA; [b] Head and Neck Surgical Associates and Oregon Health & Science University, 1849 Northwest Kearney, Suite 300, Portland, OR 97209, USA
* Corresponding author.
E-mail address: y.etan.weinstock@uth.tmc.edu

Oral Maxillofacial Surg Clin N Am 26 (2014) 151–162
http://dx.doi.org/10.1016/j.coms.2014.01.003
1042-3699/14/$ – see front matter Published by Elsevier Inc.

occur even though histopathologic evaluation of resection margins appears free of disease. There is little controversy regarding the Halsteadean notion that failure to excise all cancerous cells increases the likelihood of local or regional tumor recurrence. Therefore, our surgical ambition to clear all possible cancerous cells is appropriate, but may be incomplete.

Byers and colleagues[2] in the 1970s found a 12% local recurrence rate of oral cavity carcinomas with negative margins compared with an 80% recurrence rate with positive margins.[2] Similarly, about 5 years later, D.F.N. Harrison published a 36% rate of local recurrence of oral tongue squamous cell carcinoma (SCC) despite histologically negative margins.[3] Many more recent studies have corroborated these findings (**Table 1**). This seeming paradox indicates that local tumor recurrence patterns are multifactorial and dependent on a variety of factors rather than just the microscopic distance between normal and neoplastic tissue. Potential mechanisms include microscopic disease, field cancerization, new primaries, tumor implantation, and overall immune system failure.[4] It has been taught that minimal tissue trauma, devascularization of tumor, and negative margins were the key elements necessary to decrease the "centrifugal spread" of tumor. However, we continue to know that although negative margins may be surgically feasible, adjuvant therapy continues to be a mainstay even after adequate surgical extirpation of tumors. Despite the potential elusive mechanisms that tumors use to escape resection, leaving a positive margin decreases overall survival, even with the use of adjuvant therapy.[5,6]

ORAL CAVITY CANCER EPIDEMIOLOGY

Oral cavity SCC remains a surgical disease in the sense that the first step, and ideally the only step, necessary in its treatment is surgical extirpation. The anatomic boundaries begin at the lips and terminate at the palatoglossus and circumvallate papillae. The sites and subsites include the lips, alveolar ridge, oral tongue, floor of mouth, buccal mucosa, hard palate, and retromolar trigone. According to the National Cancer Data Base, the types of cancers involving the oral cavity include SCC (86%), adenocarcinoma (6%), verrucous carcinoma (2%), lymphoma (1.5%), and Kaposi sarcoma (1.5%).[7] The 2 preventable risk factors for SCC include tobacco (including smokeless) and alcohol. They act synergistically and increase the overall risk to 35-fold of that of controls for SCC of the oral cavity. Also, human papilloma virus (HPV) has become a new and increasing risk factor for head and neck cancer altogether. By the most recent estimates, the overall survival of oral cavity cancer has increased in the past 25 years to about 62%, 5-year related survival.[8] Some theories for the improvements include increased incidence of HPV-associated head and neck cancers, improvements in screening, and accurate staging, as well improvement in chemotherapy and radiotherapy.

MARGIN ASSESSMENT
Margin Measurements

The extent of adequate margin resection remains debatable. In 1978, Looser and colleagues[9] defined a positive surgical margin as any specimen in which invasive tumor was (1) present at the cut edge of the specimen, (2) within 5 mm of the cut edge, (3) had premalignant change at the cut edge, or (4) had in situ carcinoma at the cut edge. In general, these classic definitions have been accepted with little variation. However, early studies evaluating Mohs surgical techniques applied in oral cavity cancer resections found that 70% of 93 cases had tumor deposits located 1 cm or more away from any grossly identifiable disease. These extensions of malignant cells were able to be excised using microscopic guidance and a 91% local control rate was achieved. Conventional histologic frozen section margin assessment missed these deposits and thus a 2-cm resection margin for oral cavity cancers was proposed.[10,11] More recent studies have found that margins of less than 7 mm or depth of invasion of more than 10 mm carries a statistically significant difference in locoregional recurrence and survival.[12] The authors typically err on the side of caution and attempt 1 cm or more of visible mucosal margins and 1 cm of palpable, deep margins. Nevertheless, although this is our goal, there are multiple factors that reduce the width of the histopathologic margin from surgeon measurement.

Anatomic and Histologic Margins

Anatomic factors and tissue histology influence the ability to achieve such wide resected margins in the upper aerodigestive tract. Transoral laryngeal tumor resection studies often look at the extent of surgical margins and postsurgical outcomes. Resections of this type are often limited by the surgeon's ability to visualize and resect the entire tumor specimen transorally, thus specimens are often inherently excised piecemeal, violating the classic en bloc principle. Surgeons are also hesitant to excise critical, functional tissue close to the tumor. In these cases, margins of

Table 1
Survival rates by margin

Source	No.	Site	Positive Margin (%)	5 y Survival by Margin Status			Outcomes by Margin Status
				Clear	Close	Involved	
Patel et al,[46] 2010	547	Oral	10	80%		45	Decreased DSS if tumor is cut through (P = .09)
Kwok et al,[47] 2010	417	ORPH	13	76		58	Improved 5-y survival 72% to 76% with repeated resection
Nason et al,[48] 2009	227	Oral	22	73	62	39	Each mm of margin = 8% increased 5-y survival
Jackel et al,[49] 2007	1467	All (laser)	26	73 (LRC)	55 (LRC)	44 (LRC)	No diff. in LRC between close and involved, but clear and close with similar survival
Binahmed et al,[50] 2007	425	Oral	15	69	58	38	5-y survival better (P<.001)
Haque et al,[51] 2006	261	Larynx Oral	11	54		29	Kaiser Permanente Cancer Reg. 8-y follow-up (P = .005)
Brandwein-Gensler et al,[52] 2005	168	Oral/ORPH	22	71	18	11	No diff. in survival or L/R recurrence pattern of invasion sign
Gallo et al,[53] 2004	253	Larynx Supracricoid	16				5% vs 23% recurrence (P<.05) margin status did no predict survival
Hinerman et al,[54] 2004	226	All	30	77	86	52	Improved L/R (P<.001); no diff. overall survival
Slootweg et al,[55] 2002	394	All	47	58		34	Dutch database, 4% vs 22% local recurrence
Sessions et al,[56] 2000	235	FOM	37	71		55 (includes close)	Significant higher DSS compared with close or involved; no benefit of XRT
Jones et al,[57] 1996	352	Salvage	14	43		31	Increased local recurrence; poorer survival
Bradford et al,[58] 1996	159	Larynx	7	50	57	27	No diff. in survival or DFS
Laramore et al,[59] 1993	109	Oral/ORPH	100			29	Matched pair analysis to XRT alone = better LRC but no diff. in survival (29% vs 25%)
Loree & Strong et al,[60] 1990	398	Oral	9	60		52	L/R 36% vs 18% and significant worse survival for + margins; XRT no benefit

Abbreviations: DFS, disease-free survival; DSS, disease-specific survival; L/R, local/regional; LRC, local/regional control; ORPH, oropharynx; XRT, radiation therapy.

From Wolf GT. Surgical margins in the genomic era: The Hayes Martin Lecture, 2012. Arch Otolaryngol Head Neck Surg 2012;138(11):1001–13.

1 mm have been shown to be adequate with equivalent oncologic outcomes to wider resections, yet preserve laryngeal function.[13] One reason for this may be due to "anatomic barriers to spread" inherent in the laryngeal tissue. Within the oral cavity, many similar anatomic barriers are thought to exist. For example, SCCs of the buccal mucosa remain superficial until they reach advanced stages, whereas oral tongue SCC is more likely to invade deeply, spreading along muscle fibers, fascial planes, and lymphatics, often well beyond the region of palpable tumor. Submucosal spread of disease is also common among oropharyngeal and hypopharyngeal tumors, often precluding the ability to obtain wide 3-dimensional (3D) margins.

Biologic heterogeneity of malignant cells may also influence effects of close margins and the implications to treatment. Despite arising from the same progenitor cell, SCC arising at different subsites within the oral cavity has divergent proclivities for invasion into adjacent tissues. For example, carcinoma of the retromolar trigone certainly has a greater tendency for invasion than a carcinoma of the hard palate. This type of biologic difference also can be seen in responsiveness to radiation therapy between tumors at different oral cavity subsites.[14] These factors are important when planning your resections and orienting your specimen for pathologic assessment.

Meeting with Pathologist: Tumor Mapping

One of the more frustrating aspects of histologic assessment for pathologists is orientation of the specimen. In the current age of minimally invasive surgical approaches that may provide tumor specimens that are fragmented and not oriented, independent margin assessment is nearly impossible. Therefore, it is incumbent on the surgeon to review the specimen directly with the pathologist as soon as possible after removal to assist with accurate mapping of the tumor. This can be done by suture orientation for simple resections, or the surgeon can personally hand off the specimen to the pathologist and review the specimen orientation. This is essential in complex 3D specimens, as the specimen frequently loses clear anatomic landmark differentiation after resection. The process is identical whether the specimen was harvested via open en bloc resection or transoral robotic resection. Translating the 3D specimen into a 2D map can be difficult, and is usually aided by diagramming the specimen or photographing it (**Figs. 1** and **2**). Specimen inking also is important to clarify and differentiate the margins, especially when more than one margin is present (eg,

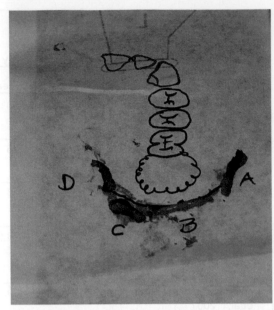

Fig. 1. A 2D map of a retromolar trigone resection with surgical margins attached. (*Courtesy of* Eric J. Dierks, MD, DMD, FACS, Portland, OR.)

superior and deep). Some surgeons elect to ink the margins themselves at the time of resection, and sterile inks are available for this purpose. Others choose to ink with the pathologist after orientation. Regardless of method, it is often helpful to maintain a good record of orientation that will be understandable to the surgeon; in the event of a positive margin, he or she can return to the appropriate wound edge for accurate reexcision. Many surgeons generate their own consistent marking methods for all cases to limit confusion and provide a consistent nomenclature (eg, short stitch = superior, long stitch = lateral).

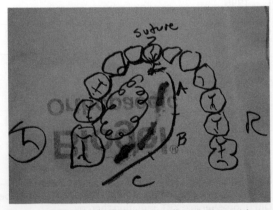

Fig. 2. A 2D map of a floor of mouth resection with surgical margins attached. (*Courtesy of* Eric J. Dierks, MD, DMD, FACS, Portland, OR.)

Moreover, one confusing issue can occur when there are intraoperative nonmargin cuts or tears. This can occur when handling this delicate tissue or an intraoperative decision to extend the resection on evaluation of the tissues. When this happens, it is advised to either repair the tissue specimen with sutures or acknowledge the tear with the pathologist and ink that region with a separate color so that it is not erroneously evaluated as the true margin. Likewise, "air margins" of tumor ulceration, particularly into the lumen of the maxillary sinus, should be clearly identified to the pathologist to avoid a false-positive margin.

Pathologic Assessment of Margins: Techniques

Once the specimen is inked and anatomically mapped with the pathologist, the specimen is often divided serially into narrow sections in a process called "bread loafing." This type of sectioning provides for "perpendicular section" of the tumor for histologic assessment of the margin from the invasive front of the tumor to the nearest edge of resection, measured in millimeters. This method has the advantage of visualizing the tumor as well as the margin edge. The bread-loaf specimen can then be frozen rapidly and the faces of the specimen sections evaluated at various levels. One inherent shortcoming of this technique is that it carries a risk of false-negative assessment because the process evaluates only representative faces of the specimen and the possibility of tumor nests extending to the edge of resection between these section faces is real. Pathologists attempt to overcome this inherent shortcoming by taking superficial and then deeper sections of each specimen slice, but this remains imprecise.

This method differs from the parallel "en face" margins taken from either the remaining tissue left behind after resection or from the tumor specimen. En face margins can allow for assessment of a greater surface area, but do not allow for evaluation of the margin width because they do not include the tumor. Both types of sections have their utility. En face margins are typically taken from the mucosal edge and can give a "yes or no" type of assessment for residual tumor. However, surgeons are more likely to have difficulty achieving clearance of tumor from the deep connective tissues rather than from the mucosal edge. This may be because of anatomic constraints or because the mucosal surface is visible and often the deep margin can be assessed surgically only by palpation. A 2005 review of histopathologic margins in oral and oropharyngeal resection specimens found that among 301 patients resected with curative intent, 70 patients were determined to have inadequate margins. Of these, 87% (61/70) involved the deep margin, whereas only 16% (11/70) involved the mucosal margins. The overall incidence of isolated positive mucosal margins was therefore a rare 2% (5/301).[15] This study also noted a higher percentage of positive margins in some oral subsites, reflecting the difficulties in excision of some regions and the anatomic barriers to spread at other sites. This finding of limited mucosal margin positivity may confound some of the newer approaches to assessment, such as confocal microscopic endoscopy or "molecular markers," which are largely limited to only the surface mucosa.

Many older publications regarding margins do not address the manner of margin assessment and it is probable that there are a combination of en face and perpendicular evaluations, thus precluding meaningful comparisons and conclusions. Because each method of margin appraisal has benefits and shortcomings, a combination approach may provide the most accurate assessment overall. This can be accomplished by excising a full-thickness en face margin circumferentially to evaluate the entire interface as well as perpendicular sections to assess margin width. However, that approach creates the potential issue of creating a fictitiously narrower margin around the tumor on perpendicular evaluation because a portion of the true margin has been sacrificed for en face review. Therefore it is imperative that any en face sample taken should be measured, notated as "off specimen" or "off patient/defect," and documented by both the pathologist and surgeon to achieve an accurate margin review.

Some debate continues over the decision to harvest margins for frozen section analysis "from the patient" or "from the specimen." Hinni and colleagues[16] noted that the submission of small tissue fragments can speed an operation and may have value in spatially complex specimens; however, his group advocated what they termed "specimen-driven" margin analysis over "defect-driven" assessment.

The different techniques of histopathologic margin assessment may be a source of surgeon frustration and may be one explanation of why intraoperative "clear" margins can become "positive" on final pathologic reporting.

Bone Margins

Oral malignancies that invade bony structures will often extend through the cortex and into the cancellous bone space where they can proliferate without significant impedance.[17] Once the cortex of the mandible is violated, the true involvement is often difficult to determine[18] and the mandibular margin is often greater than that determined by imaging techniques.[19] The high mineral content and solid structure of bone requires decalcification before it is amenable to sectioning and evaluation by traditional paraffin-embedded permanent section analysis, a process that can take days or weeks. Thus, bone margins have traditionally been determined preoperatively on imaging studies and are not readily amenable to rapid intraoperative assessment. Therefore, the need for evaluating bone margins intraoperatively for residual tumor is clear, and several studies have investigated methods for reliable assessment. Forrest and colleagues[18] evaluated cancellous bone scrapings taken from the margin edge of the remaining mandible following resection of the specimen. The scrapings were analyzed using standard frozen section technique and were later compared with the permanent decalcified bone sections to determine the predictive ability of this method. This study showed complete correlation between frozen section and the permanent specimen results. In all, 32 (97%) of 33 margins were predictive of final pathologic results with this technique. The investigators concluded that mandibular cancellous bone scraping for frozen section assessment is a strong reliable indicator of final mandibular bone margins in oral carcinoma. This technique could be used reliably for intraoperative decision making on bone margin adequacy.

Mahmood and colleagues[20] expanded on this model and performed mandibular cancellous scrapings on 7 patients undergoing segmental mandibulectomy. Their technique was different and they performed cytologic analysis of the cancellous material rather than frozen fixation, but the concept remained. They found that 14 of 14 margins examined in this fashion were correct when compared with the permanent decalcified specimens. This also showed that the predictive value and intraoperative utility of this method was inexpensive, accurate, and did not require any specialized equipment.

These techniques are limited in that they evaluate only the cancellous bone and not the cortical bone. A 2006 study by Oxford and Ducic[17] examined thin cortical scrapings taken intraoperatively by a 4-mm or 5-mm osteotome. These translucent slices are amenable to routine frozen section. They found 8 of 25 specimens were positive for malignancy at the margin edge as determined by preoperative radiologic assessment and confirmed on permanent specimen analysis. This method had an 89% (8/9) sensitivity and 100% (16/16) specificity.

Using the same concept of bone sample acquisition for margins, Wysluch and colleagues[21] examined the use of trephine drill core samples taken from the mandible in detecting metastatic disease. The investigators noted discrepancy between the frozen section and permanent section results in only 5 (6%) of 84 specimens, thereby showing a 94% consistency between the intraoperative and postoperative results. A sensitivity of 78.9% and specificity of 98.5% were calculated for this technique.

Other methods of intraoperative bone margin assessment have been proposed, including rapid microwave decalcification. Although this technique showed 100% correlation with permanent specimens, it is extremely labor intensive, taking hours to complete, and requires equipment that is not readily available in most pathology laboratories.[22]

Intraoperative assessment of bone margins can certainly be challenging; however, multiple techniques have been described that use equipment available at most institutions and exhibit excellent correlation with permanent section results. Therefore, it is our opinion that bone margins can and should be assessed during oncologic resections where bone is involved. Our method is similar to those described. We plan our resection based on preoperative imaging and typically use cancellous bone curette samples for intraoperative validation.

Tissue Shrinkage

No review of margin assessment would be complete without discussion on tissue shrinkage. Most oncologic surgeons are familiar with the frustration of performing a wide resection only to find that the tumor-free margin reported on histologic examination is significantly smaller than measured in situ. It has been described in an animal model that significant shrinkage occurs on specimens after excision with monopolar cautery. Johnson and colleagues[23] demonstrated that resected labiobuccal and tongue specimens from dogs had significant shrinkage after processing for histologic examination. The labiobuccal margin exhibited a 38.3% loss after resection with an additional 10.5% loss after fixation. The tongue margins had a 24.8% loss after resection and an additional 7.6% loss after fixation. The greatest loss occurs immediately post resection. They concluded that there is a 30% to 50% discrepancy in margins measured in situ and after processing. The shrinkage was attributed to the unopposed contractility of the underlying muscles within the specimen and the release from surrounding support structures.

In 2005, Mistry and colleagues[24] found that the mean shrinkage of tumor margins for tongue and buccal specimens in adults were 23.5% and 21.1%, respectively. The degree of tumor shrinkage was significantly less for higher-stage tumors (T3/T4: 9.2%) than for lower-stage tumors (T1/T2: 25.6%). The investigators postulated that there is loss of contractility of the resected tissues because of increased tumor involvement.

Cheng and colleagues[14] further evaluated oral tissue shrinkage and found that different oral subsites have dissimilar rates of discrepancies. In their study, buccal mucosa, mandibular alveolar ridge, and retromolar trigone tissues exhibited the greatest mean tissue shrinkage (71%) versus maxillary alveolar ridge and hard palate mucosa (53%) and oral tongue tissue (42%). In contradiction to the study by Mistry and colleagues,[24] lower-stage T1 and T2 tumors had a mean discrepancy of 51% compared with higher stages, with 75% discrepancy. This finding may be due to the increased microscopic invasiveness that is characteristic of late-stage tumors and thus decreasing the width of the palpated margin compared with the microscopic margin seen after processing.

These studies provide for generalizations that the surgeon should plan to increase the width of resection by about 25% to 50% so as to achieve a desired margin width. This concept is the basis of the perception that a 1-cm intraoperative margin should allow for more than 5-mm final margin width.

Excision Method

Numerous techniques exist for performing oral resections, including cold steel, electrocautery, carbon dioxide laser, and ultrasonic scalpel. These devices and methods have been studied and compared with regard to operative time, blood loss, wound healing, postoperative pain, and recovery times in both animal and human subjects.[25–29] There are clear data to suggest that operative time and blood loss are improved with electrosurgical techniques; however, there is sparse literature evaluating what effect each method may have on histopathologic margin assessment or tissue shrinkage. The use of energy-based devices causes some degree of tissue distortion and artifact at the surgical margin, which can potentially limit the pathologist's ability to assess adequacy. Kakarala and colleagues[30] assessed the cut specimens of resected rat tongues in a blinded fashion. The specimens were resected using either scalpel, monopolar electrocautery, or ultrasonic scalpel. The investigators found the least tissue distortion with a steel scalpel and the most distortion with monopolar electrocautery; ultrasonic scalpel distortion was intermediate. It is possible that the monopolar artifacts were overestimated in this study because of the settings used by the investigators; however, all histopathologic margin artifacts were less than 1 mm, regardless of instrument used.

George and colleagues[31] demonstrated that cold steel scalpel produced the greatest amount of tissue shrinkage, followed by ultrasonic scalpel, coagulative diathermy, and cutting diathermy, respectively, in a pig tongue model. Interestingly, control specimens of normal tongue tissue shrank more than any resection modality on processing. The investigators' hypothesis is that intact tissue causes significant tissue retraction on processing, and methods of resection that produce thermal injury to the oral tissues cause the muscle proteins to denature and therefore create less contraction and shrinkage. This notion is somewhat consistent with the study by Mistry and colleagues[24] that found less tissue shrinkage with more advanced-stage tumors compared with early-stage tumors, because in those cases the normal contractile nature of the tongue muscles is impaired. It is important to note that although statistically significant differences between modalities were seen, the actual-size discrepancies were small measurements of less than 1.5 mm for a 10-mm margin resection.

Good Margins

Because tissue shrinkage is universal, it seems incorrect to presume that the effect would cause an otherwise negative margin to become positive ex vivo. Even if it did, it seems unlikely that it would have any true prognostic significance. All studies that evaluate outcomes from oral resections with respect to margin width are subject to the same shrinkage effects, and, therefore, conclusions drawn from these remain somewhat applicable despite this issue. What remains uncertain is what constitutes a "positive" margin. The challenge is not to define an arbitrary dimensional margin measurement, but rather what represents a clinically significant or prognostically significant margin.

Margin Reporting

There is a lack of consistency among published reports with respect to marginal reporting, as there is not a universally standardized nomenclature. In the United States, synoptic tumor reporting developed by the College of American Pathologists suggests reporting the closest margin in millimeters or centimeters specifying which edge of specimen is examined. It also incorporates margin reporting if carcinoma in situ is seen near the edge of resection. It does not specifically address dysplasia at the margins. This differs from the guidelines from the Royal College of Pathologists in the United Kingdom, which classifies the margin status into 3 distinct groups: a margin greater than or equal to 5 mm is "clear," 1 to 5 mm is "close," and less than 1 mm is "involved." These traditional margin measurement cutoffs are widely accepted and used, but are somewhat arbitrary and based on studies performed more than 30 years ago that lack any current validation.[9] Additionally, viewing margin status measurements in isolation without accepting the multivariate etiology of tumorigenesis in the oral cavity seems flawed. Arbitrarily asserting that a margin smaller than 5 mm is "close" does not factor in anatomic constraints that preclude safe and justifiable tissue resection. It may be feasible to resect a 1-cm margin around a tongue base lesion, but in the buccal region, obtaining a similar margin could necessitate resection of uninvolved facial nerves and skin. That is excessive and not warranted when they are uninvolved. Also, occasionally deeper tissues beyond the resection margin are unlikely to present a barrier to tumor spread, and thus if clinically and histologically are uninvolved are likely truthfully so. Therefore, it is clear that these arbitrary measurements cannot be reliably used at all sites. These issues were nicely detailed in a recent anatomic study involving transoral cancer resections by Hinni and colleagues[32] in which it was asserted that final margin width may not be as essential as ensuring that the final inked margin is free of disease. Multiple other studies have evaluated various other margin definition cutoffs ranging from less than 2 mm to more than 10 mm, and have found varying degrees of locoregional control and disease-specific survival using these expanded margin definitions.[32–36]

Thus, we can determine that the notion of attempting 1-cm margins at all sites within the oral cavity as a surgical baseline is inherently flawed. Some may propose that in light of the availability of microvascular free tissue transfer and improved reconstructive options that wide resection margins of a specific dimension should routinely be taken. However, this practice has not been shown to affect prognosis. Additionally, molecular markers have shown that even "clear" margins on histopathologic review show evidence of genetic changes in the residual mucosa that increase risks of local recurrence.[14] This field cancerization concept suggests that despite our best attempts at obtaining negative surgical margins of any dimension, patients may develop recurrent tumors.

THERAPEUTIC IMPLICATIONS OF POSITIVE MARGINS

There is little consensus in the literature regarding appropriate management of positive margins. For regions in the oral cavity that are easily accessible and amenable to reexcision, many surgeons may opt to attempt repeat resection. However, identification of the positive margin region after an en bloc resection can be difficult and is often imprecise. Partial glossectomy surgery is exemplary of this problem. Consider a tongue resection in which the size of the surgical defect is larger than the initial outlined excision due to shrinkage that occurs on the residual tongue and not just the specimen; direct correlation from tumor to remnant is difficult. Additionally, because the remaining tongue muscles are oriented in various directions and have different amounts of retraction based on their native contractility, the exposed resection face may not contain the true margin of resection and there is no way to determine the extent of re-resection required to eradicate all malignant cells. It is common that reexcision after obtaining a positive margin will not yield any residual tumor; however, that does not invalidate this approach.[33]

Because we can assert that a truly positive "cut-through" margin can leave remnant carcinoma behind despite re-resection attempts, and histologically positive surgical margins confer a worse prognosis, the addition of adjuvant therapies in the face of a positive resection margin has been widely studied.[37] Multiple publications have shown that the addition of chemotherapy to adjuvant radiotherapy improves locoregional control and improved overall survival in high-risk patients after surgery when margins are concerning. In 2 large, prospective, randomized trials, these high-risk factors were described as "positive margins"; however, these were generalized as "less than 5 mm" and "at the surgical margin."[5,6] Although the benefit of combined modality therapy for "positive margins" is clear, the nonstandardized margin reporting underscores the need for consistency to guide postoperative decision making.

Another problematic issue is the effect of field cancerization on margin status. This may lead to dysplasia at the margin edge; however, the entire region surrounding the resection must be considered to have similar mucosal change. Thus, there is currently no guideline to determine the extent or clinical impact of further resection in this setting.

FUTURE DIRECTIONS

If the concept of "clear" margins in fact does reduce the local and regional recurrence despite adjuvant therapy, we need to develop new techniques to identify the molecular margin. We know from tumor biology that genetic alterations are what drive tumorigenesis. Thus, there are genetic alterations that occur well before the phenotypic manifestation can occur. Therefore, tissue may grossly and microscopically appear normal at the margins, but indeed positive molecular margins remain. If these molecular margins could be found intraoperatively, it may lead the surgeon to pursue further resection or a more aggressive adjuvant avenue after gross resection. Also, after resection with or without adjuvant therapy, there remains the risk of recurrence. Methods of early detection other than physical examination and diagnostic imaging may lead to earlier treatment of recurrence.

Two fairly new concepts could answer these questions and lead to advances of earlier detection: adequate margin assessment and improved surveillance. One method includes the utility of epigenetic markers and the other includes the utility of optical imaging and autofluorescence.

Epigenetics refers to the study of changes in gene expression. We have a plethora of knowledge over the past decades that have described the errors and expression changes that occur in cancer. Tumor-suppressor genes, proto-oncogenes and promoter sequence hypermethylation are hallmarks of tumor biology. Most notably, p53, or "guardian of the genome" has been implicated in mostly all kinds of malignancies, but is present in less than 50% of HNSCC.[38,39] Therefore, as the research has continued in epigenetics, more and more HNSCC-specific markers have been identified. Most of the markers identified were found to have hypermethylation of promoter sequences, rendering them inactive. For example, p16 is a cyclin-dependent kinase that regulates cell cycle and when rendered inactive, triggers a cascade of events that eventually leads to malignancy. Because methylation is a key component of these alterations, identifying these hypermethylated sequences serves as markers for aberrant genetic transformation. In the past, these methylation studies were time consuming; however, Goldenberg and colleagues in 2004[40] published their results on the quantitative methylation-specific polymerase chain reaction protocol and found that this technique is feasible and can be performed intraoperatively. Specifically, Shaw and colleagues in 2007[41] used methylation assays for p16 and cytoglobin and found 65% positive margins and 46% recurrence out of those specimens with positive margins. Moreover, other studies have examined more aberrantly methylated gene-promoters. In 2011, Supic and colleagues[42] examined aberrant hypermethylation of p16, DAPK, RASSF1A, APC, WIF1, RUNX3, E-cad, MGMT, and hMLH1 genes in histologically negative surgical margins of patients with oral SCC. Their conclusion was that out of all markers examined, DAPK hypermethylation was associated with decreased survival; this was statistically significant. The development of a cocktail of sequences that can be readily available intraoperatively and that can be quickly assessed could lead surgeons to resect more if possible. Otherwise, if further resection is technically not feasible or leads to mutilation, the surgeon may pursue aggressive adjuvant avenues after surgical resection of the obvious disease to halt the altered molecular march.

On the other hand, new concepts in autofluorescent imaging and optical imaging also have been studied as adjuncts to noninvasively ascertaining malignant transformation. Autofluorescent imaging illuminates tissue using near-ultraviolet light; this is captured by camera or eye. The tissue illuminates to various degrees, especially the stroma and collagen. As dysplastic and neoplastic transformation occurs, there is a decrease in collagen and an overall increase in epithelial thickening, thus decreasing the autofluorescent illumination.[43] Autofluorescent imaging was borne out of photodynamic therapy. Its use for neoplasia began in the 1970s. Studies in the 1990s and early 2000s have shown its increased presence in the clinic as a screening tool; however, the sensitivity and specificity remain questionable. Awan and colleagues in 2011[44] found in 126 patients the sensitivity and specificity to be 84% and 15%, respectively. Its utility for margin assessment remains questionable because its comparison is standard hematoxylin and eosin pathology sections. However, it is gaining increased notoriety at the clinic level. A newer optical imaging tool, high-resolution microendoscopy (HRME), uses a topical fluorescent agent and an HRME optic probe to examine questionable sites in the oral cavity for microscopic margin assessment. Its accuracy has been studied recently and this tool was able to detect a wide range of abnormal tissue from mild to moderate dysplasia and cancer. Its sensitivity and specificity were 93% and 96%, respectively.[45] The prospect of using a noninvasive instrument to identify the dysplastic front in vivo during surgery to guide surgical margins is very enticing.

We currently do not use these methods in our practice, but one could see the potential on the horizon. Ideally, if these methods were easily and readily reproduced, they would theoretically allow precise margin assessment down to the genetic level and also allow for painless and accurate assessment of dysplastic changes during surveillance.

SUMMARY

The only factor that the oncologic surgeon can control in management of oral malignancy is the extent of resection and the surgical margin. However, it is clear that despite the surgeon's best efforts and seemingly wide and "adequate" resections, margin status may be narrower than anticipated and recurrence is possible, regardless. Incomplete tumor resections negatively affect prognosis and therefore surgeons must strive to obtain negative surgical margins in all cases. There are limitations in tissue factors and specimen evaluation that can affect the ability to obtain "clear" margins; however, the definitions and implications of these margins are evolving as we develop greater understanding of the nuances of malignancies within the oral cavity. Future directions will allow for a rapid and reliable, accurate assessment of the margins on a molecular level to guide precise excision. Until then, we must continue to be diligent with our preoperative assessment, conservative yet accurate with our intraoperative margins, and maintain a close relationship with our pathologists.

REFERENCES

1. Jesse RH, Sugarbaker EV. Squamous cell carcinoma of the oropharynx: why we fail. Am J Surg 1976;132:435–8.
2. Byers RM, Bland KI, Borlase B, et al. The prognostic and therapeutic value of frozen section determinations in the surgical treatment of squamous carcinoma of the head and neck. Am J Surg 1978;136:525–8.
3. Harrison D. The questionable value of total glossectomy. Head Neck Surg 1983;6:632–8.
4. Wolf GT. Surgical margins in the genomic era: The Hayes Martin Lecture, 2012. Arch Otolaryngol Head Neck Surg 2012;11:1001–13.
5. Cooper JS, Pajak TF, Forastiere AA, et al, Radiation Therapy Oncology Group 9501/Intergroup. Postoperative concurrent radiotherapy and chemotherapy for high-risk squamous-cell carcinoma of the head and neck. N Engl J Med 2004;350(19):1937–44.
6. Bernier J, Domenge C, Ozsahin M, et al, European Organziation for Research Treatment of Cancer Trial 22931. Postoperative irradiation with or without concomitant chemotherapy for locally advanced head and neck cancer. N Engl J Med 2004; 350(19):1945–52.
7. Hoffman HT, Karnell LH, Funk GF, et al. The National Cancer Data Base report on cancer of the head and neck. Arch Otolaryngol Head Neck Surg 1998;124:951–62.
8. Pulte D, Brenner H. Changes in survival in head and neck cancers in the late 20th and early 21st century: a period analysis. Oncologist 2010;15:994–1001.
9. Looser KG, Shah JP, Strong EW. The significance of "positive" margins in surgically resected epidermoid carcinomas. Head Neck Surg 1978;1:107–11.
10. Davidson TM, Nahum AM, Astarita RW. Microscopic controlled excisions for epidermoid carcinoma of the head and neck. Otolaryngol Head Neck Surg 1981;89(2):244–51.
11. Davidson TM, Haghighi P, Astarita R, et al. Microscopically oriented histologic surgery for head and neck mucosal cancer. Cancer 1987;60(8):1856–61.
12. Liao CT, Huang SF, Chen IH, et al. When does skin excision allow the achievement of an adequate local control rate in patients with squamous cell carcinoma involving the buccal mucosa? Ann Surg Oncol 2008;15(8):2187–94.
13. Grant DG, Bradley PT, Parmar A, et al. Implications of positive margins or incomplete excision in laryngeal cancer treated by transoral laser microsurgery: how we do it. Clin Otolaryngol 2009;34:485–9.
14. Cheng A, Cox D, Schmidt BL. Oral squamous cell carcinoma margin discrepancy after resection and pathologic processing. J Oral Maxillofac Surg 2008;66:523–9.
15. Woolgar JA, Triantafyllou A. A histopathological appraisal of surgical margins in oral and oropharyngeal cancer resection specimens. Oral Oncol 2005;41:1034–43.
16. Hinni ML, Ferlito A, Brandwein-Gensler MS, et al. Surgical margins in head and neck cancer: a contemporary review. Head Neck 2013;35:1362–70.
17. Oxford LE, Ducic Y. Intraoperative evaluation of cortical bony margins with frozen section analysis. Otolaryngol Head Neck Surg 2006;134:138–41.
18. Forrest LA, Schuller DE, Lucas JG, et al. Rapid analysis of mandibular margins. Laryngoscope 1995;105:475–7.
19. Totsuka Y, Usui Y, Tei K, et al. Mandibular involvement by squamous cell carcinoma of the lower alveolus: analysis and comparative study of histologic and radiographic features. Head Neck Surg 1991;13:40–50.
20. Mahmood S, Conway D, Ramesar KC. Use of intraoperative cytologic assessment of mandibular marrow scrapings to predict resection margin status in patients with squamous cell carcinoma. J Oral Maxillofac Surg 2001;59:1138–41.

21. Wysluch A, Stricker I, Holzle F, et al. Intraoperative evaluation of bony margins with frozen-section analysis and trephine drill extraction technique: a preliminary study. Head Neck 2010;32:1473–8.

22. Weisberger EC, Hillburn M, Johnson B, et al. Intra-operative microwave processing of bone margins during resection of head and neck cancer. Arch Otolaryngol Head Neck Surg 2001;127:790–3.

23. Johnson RE, Sigman JD, Funk GF, et al. Quantification of surgical margin shrinkage in the oral cavity. Head Neck 1997;19:281–6.

24. Mistry RC, Qureshi SS, Kumaran C. Post-resection mucosal margin shrinkage in oral cancer: quantification and significance. J Surg Oncol 2005;91:131–3.

25. Basu MK, Frame JW, Rhys Evans PH. Wound healing following partial glossectomy using the CO2 laser, diathermy and scalpel: a histological study in rats. J Laryngol Otol 1988;102:322–7.

26. Liboon J, Funkhouser W, Terris DJ. A comparison of mucosal incisions made by scalpel, CO2 laser, electrocautery, and constant-voltage electrocautery. Otolaryngol Head Neck Surg 1997;116:379–85.

27. Chinpairoj S, Feldman M, Saunders JC, et al. A comparison of monopolar electrosurgery to a new multipolar electrosurgical system in a rat model. Laryngoscope 2001;111:213–7.

28. Sinha UK, Gallagher LA. Effects of steel scalpel, ultrasonic scalpel, CO2 laser, and monopolar and bipolar electrosurgery on wound healing in guinea pig oral mucosa. Laryngoscope 2003;113:228–36.

29. Metternich FU, Wenzel S, Sagowski C, et al. The "Ultracision Harmonic Scalpel" ultrasound activated scalpel. Initial results in surgery of the tongue and soft palate. HNO 2002;50:733–8.

30. Kakarala K, Faquin WC, Deschler DG. Effect of glossectomy technique on histopathologic assessment in a rat model. Head Neck 2011;33:1576–80.

31. George KS, Hyde NC, Wilson P, et al. Does the method of resection affect the margins of tumours in the oral cavity? Prospective controlled study in pigs. Br J Oral Maxillofac Surg 2013;51(7):600–3.

32. Hinni ML, Zarka MA, Hoxworth JM. Margin mapping in transoral surgery for head and neck cancer. Laryngoscope 2013;123:1190–8.

33. Amaral TM, Freire AR, Carvalho AL, et al. Predictive factors of occult metastasis and prognosis of clinical stages I and II squamous cell carcinoma of the tongue and floor of mouth. Oral Oncol 2004;40:780–6.

34. Weijers M, Snow GB, Bezemer DP, et al. The status of the deep surgical margins in tongue and floor of mouth squamous cell carcinoma and risk of local recurrence: an analysis of 68 patients. Int J Oral Maxillofac Surg 2004;33:146–9.

35. Brandwein-Gensler M, Teixeira MS, Lewis CM, et al. Oral squamous cell carcinoma: histologic risk assessment, but not margin status, is strongly predictive of local disease-free and overall survival. Am J Surg Pathol 2005;29:167–78.

36. Wong LS, McMahon J, Devine J, et al. Influence of close resection margins on local recurrence and disease-specific survival in oral and oropharyngeal carcinoma. Br J Oral Maxillofac Surg 2012;50:102–8.

37. Patel RS, Goldstein DP, Guillemaud J, et al. Impact of positive frozen section microscopic tumor cut-through revised to negative on oral carcinoma control and survival rates. Head Neck 2010;32:1444–51.

38. Boyle JO, Hakim J, Koch W, et al. The incidence of p53 mutations increases with progression of Head and neck cancer. Cancer Res 1993;53:4477–80.

39. Maestro R, Dolcetti R, Gasparotto D, et al. High frequency of p53 gene alteration sassociated with protein overexpression in human squamous cell carcinoma of the larynx. Oncogene 1992;7:1159–66.

40. Goldenberg D, Harden S, Masayesva BG, et al. Intraoperative molecular margin analysis in head and neck cancer. Arch Otolaryngol Head Neck Surg 2004;130:39–44.

41. Shaw RJ, Hall GL, Woolgar JA, et al. Quantitative methylation analysis of resection margins and lymph nodes in oral squamous cell carcinoma. Br J Oral Maxillofac Surg 2007;45(8):617–22.

42. Supic G, Kozomara R, Jovic N, et al. Prognostic significance of tumor-related genes hypermethylation detected in cancer-free surgical margins of oral squamous cell carcinomas. Oral Oncol 2011;47:702–8.

43. De Veld DC, Witjes MJ, Sterenborg HJ, et al. The status of in vivo autofluorescence spectroscopy and imaging for oral oncology. Oral Oncol 2005;41:117–31.

44. Awan KH, Morgan PR, Warnakulasuriya S. Evaluation of an autofluorescence based imaging system (VELscope™) in the detection of oral potentially malignant disorders and benign keratoses. Oral Oncol 2011;47:274–7.

45. Pierce MC, Schwarz RA, Bhattar VS. Accuracy of in vivo multimodal optical imaging for detection of oral neoplasia. Cancer Prev Res 2012;5:801–9.

46. Patel RS, Goldstein DP, Guillemaud J, et al. Impact of positive frozen section microscopic tumor cut-through revised to negative on oral carcinoma control and survival rates. Head Neck 2010;32(11):1444–51.

47. Kwok P, Gleich O, Hübner G, et al. Prognostic importance of "clear versus revised margins" in oral and oropharyngeal cancer. Head Neck 2010;32(11):1479–84.

48. Nason RW, Binahmed A, Pathak KA, et al. What is the adequate margin of surgical resection in oral cancer? Oral Surg Oral Med Oral Pathol Oral Radiol Endod 2009;107(5):625–9.

49. Jackel MC, Ambrosch P, Martin A, et al. Impact of re-resection for inadequate margins on the prognosis of upper aerodigestive tract cancer treated by laser microsurgery. Laryngoscope 2007; 117(2):350–6.

50. Binahmed A, Nason RW, Abdoh AA. The clinical significance of the positive surgical margin in oral cancer. Oral Oncol 2007;43(8):780–4.

51. Haque R, Contreras R, McNicoll MP, et al. Surgical margins and survival after head and neck cancer survey. BMC Ear Nose Throat Disord 2006;6:2.

52. Brandwein-Gensler M, Teixeira MS, Lewis CM, et al. Oral squamous cell carcinoma: histologic risk assessment, but not margin status, is strongly predictive of local disease-free and overall survival. Am J Surg Pathol 2005;29(2):167–8.

53. Gallo A, Manciocco V, Tropiano ML, et al. Prognostic value of resection margins in supracricoid laryngectomy. Laryngoscope 2004;114(4):616–21.

54. Hinerman RW, Mendenhall WM, Morris CG, et al. Postoperative irradiation for squamous cell carcinoma of oral cavity: 35-year experience. Head Neck 2004;26(11):984–94.

55. Slootweg PJ, Hordijk GJ, Schade Y, et al. Treatment failure and margin status in head and neck cancer: a critical view on the potential value of molecular pathology. Oral Oncol 2002;38(5):500–3.

56. Sessions DG, Spector GJ, Lenox J, et al. Analysis of treatment results for floor-of-mouth cancer. Laryngoscope 2000;110(10 Pt 1):1764–72.

57. Jones AS, Bin Hanafi Z, Nadapalan V, et al. Do positive resection margins after ablative surgery for head and neck cancer adversely affect prognosis? A study of 352 patients with recurrent carcinoma following radiotherapy treated by salvage surgery. Br J Cancer 1996;74(1):128–32.

58. Bradford CR, Wolf GT, Fisher SG, et al. Prognostic importance of surgical margins in advanced laryngeal squamous carcinoma. Head Neck 1996;18(1):11–6.

59. Laramore GE, Scott CB, Schuller DE, et al. Is a surgical resection leaving positive margins of benefit to the patient with locally advanced squamous cell carcinoma of the head and neck: a comparative study using the intergroup study 0034 and Radiation Therapy Oncology Group head and neck dataase. Int J Radiat Oncol Biol Phys 1993;27(5):1011–6.

60. Loree TR, Strong EW. Significance of positive margins in oral cavity squamous carcinoma. Am J Surg 1990;160(4):410–4.

Chemotherapy for Oral and Maxillofacial Tumors: An Update

Ahmed Eid, MD[a],*, Shuang Li, MD[b], Rodolfo Garza, DDS[c],
Mark E. Wong, DDS[c]

KEYWORDS

- Chemotherapy • Locally advanced • Maxillofacial tumors • Oral cavity tumors
- Squamous cell carcinoma

KEY POINTS

- Surgery has always been the primary intervention in oral and maxillofacial tumors and under ideal circumstances is curative.
- Squamous cell carcinoma Is by far the most common histologic subtype of head and neck tumors, including oral and maxillofacial tumors. Therefore, the results of chemotherapy trials for head and neck cancer are likely to be applicable to oral and maxillofacial cancers too, despite the lack of studies on these tumors specifically.
- There is no evidence to support the use of induction or adjuvant chemotherapy in the initial therapy of early-stage oral and maxillofacial tumors.
- Locally advanced tumors, nonresectable tumors, as well as recurrence in early-stage disease need a multimodality therapeutic approach involving chemotherapy.
- Palliative chemotherapy plays an important role in the treatment of patients with metastatic oral and maxillofacial tumors.
- Chemotherapy and targeted agents play an important role in the treatment of patients with rare oral and maxillofacial tumors, such as sarcomas, lymphomas, and giant cell tumors.

There will be more than approximately 25,000 new cases of oral cavity tumors involving the mouth and tongue in 2013 according to the American Cancer Society.[1] Early-stage oral and maxillofacial tumors—those that are less than or equal to 4 cm in greatest diameter and that do not invade surrounding structures or involve lymph nodes— account for 30% to 40% of these tumors and are usually treated with either surgery or radiation alone; this patient group has a 5-year overall survival (OS) rate exceeding 80%. Roughly 50% of patients present with locally advanced disease, which requires a multimodal approach. The remaining 10% to 20% of patients present with recurrent or metastatic disease with a 5-year survival rate dropping to less than 30%, and therapy is considered only palliative.[2]

Squamous cell carcinoma (SCC) is by far the most common histologic subtype of head and neck tumors, including oral and maxillofacial tumors. Therefore, the results of chemotherapy trials for head and neck cancer are likely to be applicable to oral and maxillofacial cancers too, despite the lack of studies on these tumors specifically. The focus of this article is to review the role of chemotherapy in the treatment of these

Disclosures: None.
[a] Department of General Oncology, The University of Texas MD Anderson Cancer Center, 1515 Holcombe Boulevard, Unit 0462, Houston, TX 77030, USA; [b] Internal Medicine, University of Texas Health Science Center at Houston, 6431 Fannin, Houston, TX 77030, USA; [c] Oral & Maxillofacial Surgery, University of Texas Health Science Center at Houston, 6516 MD Anderson Boulevard, Houston, TX 77030, USA
* Corresponding author.
E-mail address: aeid@mdanderson.org

Oral Maxillofacial Surg Clin N Am 26 (2014) 163–169
http://dx.doi.org/10.1016/j.coms.2014.01.004
1042-3699/14/$ – see front matter © 2014 Elsevier Inc. All rights reserved.

complex cancers including rare oral and maxillo-facial tumors, such as sarcomas, lymphomas, and giant cell tumors. The current recommendations are reviewed and new modalities are explored. A shared understanding of what is available today and perhaps in the near future will allow surgeons and medical and radiation oncologists to provide the best care for their patients.

CHEMOTHERAPY FOR EARLY-STAGE DISEASE

There is no evidence to support the use of induction or adjuvant chemotherapy as part of the initial management of these patients. These tumors are treated with surgery or radiation alone, which is often curative.

CHEMOTHERAPY FOR LOCALLY ADVANCED RESECTABLE DISEASE
Role of Neoadjuvant Chemotherapy

For locally advanced resectable tumors, only one-half of these patients are cured using surgery or radiation alone.[3] There has thus been interest in neoadjuvant and adjuvant chemotherapy to reduce these recurrences. A 2003 study of 195 patients by Licitra and colleagues[4] was randomized to receive 3 cycles of cisplatin and fluorouracil (5-FU) followed by surgery or surgery alone for resectable, early-stage (T2-T4) SCCs of the oral cavity. The 5-year OS rate did not differ significantly between the 2 arms. However, those who received neoadjuvant chemotherapy were less likely to need mandibulectomy and/or radiation.

In a more recent study, Zhong and colleagues[5] conducted a randomized phase III trial to investigate whether 2 cycles of induction docetaxel, cisplatin, and 5-FU followed by surgery and post-operative radiation were superior to surgery alone followed by postoperative radiation in patients with resectable stage III/IVA oral SCCs. Although the 2 arms did not differ significantly in OS, the induction therapy arm did show a nonsignificant trend toward a lower incidence of distant metastasis than the other arm, which was not the primary end point of the trial. Patients who received induction chemotherapy and had a favorable pathologic or clinical response had a decreased risk for death and recurrence compared with the surgery followed by postoperative radiation arm. In addition, a lower risk for death and longer distant metastasis-free survival was observed in clinical N2 patients treated with induction chemotherapy compared with the surgery followed by postoperative radiation arm.

Although these trials did not focus specifically on oral and maxillofacial tumors, their findings regarding induction chemotherapy are generally disappointing.

Role of Adjuvant Chemotherapy

The risk of recurrence after resection is significantly greater if the resected specimen reveals tumor cells extending beyond the lymph node capsule or capsules (ie, extracapsular extension [ECE]) or positive resection margins.[6]

In these situations, adding adjuvant chemotherapy concurrently with radiation therapy after surgical resection has been shown to improve treatment outcomes. In a 2004 study by Bernier and colleagues,[7] patients with risk factors for recurrence who had undergone resection and had no distant metastasis randomly received either concurrent radiation (66 Gy over a period of 6.5 weeks) therapy and cisplatin (100 mg/m^2 on days 1, 22, and 43 after resection) or the same radiation therapy alone. The median progression-free survival (PFS) was superior for the combined approach, particularly in patients who had positive margins and/or ECE: 55 months, compared with 23 months for radiation alone. However, the addition of cisplatin did not benefit patients whose tumors had vascular emboli or perineural invasion, or those who had local spread to 2 or more lymph nodes.

CHEMOTHERAPY FOR LOCALLY ADVANCED UNRESECTABLE DISEASE

The goal of chemotherapy in patients with locally advanced oral and maxillofacial cancers is to shrink the tumor sufficiently to enable surgical resection or to treat those that do not qualify for surgery at all.

Induction Chemotherapy Before Radiation Versus Radiation

Studies have shown the benefits of platinum-based induction chemotherapy in SCC in locally advanced unresectable disease. Paccagnella and colleagues[8] showed that patients with either stage III or IV SCC tumors without distant metastatic disease who were not candidates for surgery had a 21% OS rate at 5 years when they underwent 4 cycles of neoadjuvant cisplatin and 5-FU followed by radiotherapy as opposed to an 8% OS rate in similar patients who received radiotherapy alone. The participants of the study who were deemed resectable after treatment and underwent surgical resection did not have any survival benefit with the addition of chemotherapy.

Induction Chemotherapy Before Concurrent Chemoradiation

Adding taxanes to platinum-containing induction chemotherapy regimens has also been shown to have benefit. Posner and colleagues[9] showed a median survival of 71 months when docetaxel was added to a regimen of cisplatin and 5-FU for patients with stage III or IV SCC of the oral cavity, larynx, oropharynx, or hypopharynx that were unresectable and had no evidence of metastatic disease compared with median survival of 30 months for cisplatin and 5-FU alone. Both arms were subsequently treated with carboplatin-based chemoradiotherapy. The addition of docetaxel also led to a lower rate of regional recurrence, although the rate of distant metastasis was not affected. These findings were reinforced by Vermorken and colleagues,[10] who performed a similar study in which patients with stage III or IV SCC disease of the head and neck without evidence of metastasis received docetaxel and cisplatin (day 1) plus continuous infusion 5-FU (days 1–5) or cisplatin and 5-FU every 3 weeks for 4 cycles. Both arms subsequently received radiotherapy. For the taxane group (ie, those who received docetaxel), the median PFS was 11 months and the median OS was 18.8 months, whereas for the nontaxane group, the median PFS was 8.2 months and the median OS was 14.5 months.

In the highly anticipated phase III, multicenter, international trial (DeCIDE [Docetaxel Based Chemotherapy Plus or Minus Induction Chemotherapy to Decrease Events in Head and Neck Cancer]), patients with stage N2 or N3 SCC without metastasis and were treatment-naive were randomized to receive either concurrent chemoradiation with docetaxel (25 mg/m^2), continuous infusion 5-FU, and hydroxyurea (Hydrea) immediately preceding hyperfractionated radiation twice daily (150 cGy/fraction) or 2 cycles of induction chemotherapy with docetaxel (75 mg/m^2), cisplatin (75 mg/m^2), and continuous 5-FU followed by the same regimen of radiotherapy. No significant differences in OS were found between the 2 trial arms. However, the induction chemotherapy arm of the trial had a significantly lower cumulative incidence of distant metastasis. Why this result did not translate into improved OS is unclear. A possible explanation is that the trial accrued only 280 of the 400 patients that were originally planned.[11] The PARADIGM (Combination Chemotherapy and Radiation in Treating Patients With Stage III or IV Head and Neck Cancer) trial, another phase III randomized trial, enrolled patients with locally advanced head and neck cancers (55%

oropharynx, 16% larynx, 11% hypopharynx, and 18% oral cavity). Patients were treated with either docetaxel, cisplatin, and 5-FU induction therapy or concurrent cisplatin chemoradiation.[12] As in the DeCIDE trial, OS did not differ significantly between the 2 treatment arms. However, as with the prior study, this trial also did not accrue the planned number of patients.

Role of Epidermal Growth Factor Inhibitors

In a 2006 study comparing the combination of the epidermal growth factor receptor (EGFR) monoclonal antibody cetuximab and radiation with radiation alone for locoregionally advanced SCC of the head and neck, Bonner and colleagues[13] found that patients in the combination treatment arm had a median OS of 49 months, whereas those receiving radiation alone had a median OS of 29.3 months. Importantly, the addition of cetuximab did not increase systemic toxicity. At 5 years of follow-up, survival was 45.6% for the combination group and 36.4% for radiation alone.

Although cetuximab in addition to radiation is superior to radiation alone, the addition of cetuximab to cisplatin-based chemotherapy has not proven to be beneficial.[14]

CHEMOTHERAPY FOR METASTATIC OR RECURRENT DISEASE

Although many patients with locally advanced oral cavity tumors respond to treatment and can be cured, others experience recurrence. Treatment options for patients with persistent or recurrent disease that is not resectable are similar to those for patients who present with metastatic disease. For both groups of patients, the focus of therapy shifts from cure to prolonging survival and maintaining good quality of life. In deciding whether to treat a patient with recurrent or persistent residual disease that is not resectable and how to treat, clinicians must consider the patient's performance status (PS). Using the Eastern Cooperative Oncology Group grading of PS,[15] a patient with a PS of 0 to 1 may tolerate combination chemotherapy with cisplatin, 5-FU, and cetuximab, whereas those with poorer PS are conventionally treated with single-agent therapy involving 5-FU, platinum agents, taxanes, methotrexate, or Cetuximab.

Cytotoxic Chemotherapy

Platinum-based chemotherapy consisting of either cisplatin or carboplatin is the usual first-line treatment for inoperable recurrent or metastatic SCC of the head and neck. Many studies were performed to compare the efficacy of single-agent chemotherapy to combination regimens. Forastiere and colleagues[16] compared single-agent methotrexate with a combination of cisplatin or carboplatin plus 5-FU for metastatic SCC of the head and neck and found higher response rates in patients treated with platinum agents plus 5-FU than in those treated with methotrexate alone. However, the combination of platinum agents and 5-FU resulted in increased toxicity without any improvement in OS. Jacobs and colleagues[17] compared cisplatin alone, 5-FU alone, and the combination of the 2 in patients with recurrent head and neck SCC. They also concluded no OS benefit. Of the 249 patients in the study, 104 had primary SCC of the oral cavity, and all had a PS less than 4. Gibson and colleagues[18] compared a combination of cisplatin/5-FU to an alternative combination of cisplatin/paclitaxel in 218 patients with locally advanced, recurrent, or metastatic SCC of the head and neck. Forty-four patients had primary oral cavity SCC, and all patients in the study had a PS less than 3. Gibson also failed to find a significant difference between treatment arms in response rate or OS.

Targeted Therapy

In recent years, research in head and neck therapy has shifted to targeted therapies. In 1993, Dassonville and colleagues[19] found detectable EGFR expression in almost all head and neck SCCs. This EGFR overexpression was associated with shorter relapse-free time and shorter OS. These and subsequent findings led to interest in therapies targeting EGFR (cetuximab) in patients with head and neck tumors. The 2008 EXTREME (Cetuximab (Erbitux) in Combination With Cisplatin or Carboplatin and 5-Fluorouracil in the First Line Treatment of Subjects With Recurrent and/or Metastatic Squamous Cell Carcinoma of the Head and Neck) trial, conducted by Vermorken and colleagues,[20] studied patients with recurrent and metastatic SCC of the head or neck who received either combination cisplatin/5-FU or combination cisplatin/5-FU/cetuximab. Of the 442 patients, only 88 had oral cavity primary tumors. The median OS duration was 10.1 months for those who received cetuximab in contrast to 7.4 months for those who did not receive cetuximab. Similarly, those who received cetuximab had a median PFS of 5.6 months in contrast to 3.3 months for those who did not. Although no cetuximab-related deaths occurred, there was a higher incidence of sepsis in the cetuximab group than in the other group. Rates of anemia, neutropenia, and thrombocytopenia did not differ between the

2 treatment arms. The authors concluded that adding cetuximab to platinum-based chemotherapy with 5-FU significantly improved OS and response rate when given as first-line treatment. The activity of single-agent Cetuximab was illustrated by a series of 103 patients with progressive disease following platinum-based therapy.[21]

Although still in the very early stages of investigation, the EGFR tyrosine kinase inhibitor erlotinib has also been shown to be well tolerated in patients with recurrent/metastatic head and neck SCC by Kim and colleagues[22] in a phase II study. Forty-three patients with PS less than 3 had median OS of 11 months and PFS of 6 months at a follow-up time of 19 months. A monoclonal antibody that targets vascular endothelial growth factor (VEGF), bevacizumab (Avastin), is currently undergoing clinical trials in patients with recurrent or metastatic SCC of the head and neck because it has demonstrated activity in several solid tumors, such as colon, lung, and kidney. It has been demonstrated that VEGF signaling is upregulated by EGFR expression[23] and it is also hypothesized that EGFR inhibition has an anti-angiogenic effect and down-regulates VEGF.[24] Thus, combination therapy may offer benefit in metastatic SCC. Early results of an ongoing phase II trial by Argiris and colleagues[25] show that combination bevacizumab/cetuximab resulted in median PFS of 2.8 months and OS of 7.5 months.

RARE TUMORS

Other rare tumors, such as osteosarcoma, lymphoma, and giant cell tumor, can manifest themselves in the maxilla and mandible as well. Because of the rarity of these tumors in the oral and maxillofacial region, treatment is based mostly on the treatments used for these tumors at other sites of the body.

Osteosarcoma

In general, 5% to 13% of all cases of osteosarcoma occur in the jaws. DeAngelis and colleagues[26] studied osteosarcoma of the head and neck. Their study was a cohort in which 15 cases were studied (14 primary cases and 1 locally recurrent case). The mandible and maxilla were equally affected with a predilection for posterior sites. Three patients received neoadjuvant chemotherapy followed by surgery; 5 patients received surgery followed by adjuvant chemotherapy; 4 patients received a combination of both neoadjuvant and adjuvant chemotherapy, and 3 patients received no chemotherapy. Various combinations of cisplatin, doxorubicin (Adriamycin), methotrexate, ifosfamide, and etoposide were used. Extensive tumor necrosis was seen in only 1 of the 7 patients who received neoadjuvant chemotherapy. Neoadjuvant chemotherapy, adjuvant chemotherapy, and a combination of the 2 were not found to affect survival significantly. Disease-free survival rate at 15 years was 74%. The poor response to chemotherapy may have been due to the small sample size, positive resection margins, or large tumor size.

Dhima and colleagues[27] reported on the treatment of one patient with a high-grade osteoblastic osteosarcoma of the mandible (grade 3 or 4) using a neoadjuvant chemotherapy protocol similar to that of the international European and American Osteosarcoma Study Group trial. Treatment began with 3 cycles of doxorubicin, cisplatin, and high-dose methotrexate, which produced an excellent tumor response before subtotal mandibulectomy. After surgical recovery, one cycle of doxorubicin and cisplatin was administered followed by 2 cycles of high-dose methotrexate. Examinations were performed every 4 months and consisted of bone scans, chest radiography, computed tomography of the chest, and magnetic resonance imaging of the head and neck. The patient was disease-free at 25-month follow-up. The most important factor for treating osteosarcoma seems to be adequate initial resection.

Lymphoma

Another tumor that can manifest itself in the maxilla or mandible is non-Hodgkin's lymphoma. Pazoki and colleagues[28] presented 4 cases in which chemotherapy treatment produced promising results. Two of the patients were treated with a combination of local radiation and the CHOP (cyclophosphamide, hydroxydoxorubicin, vincristine, and prednisone) regimen, and the other 2 patients were treated with CHOP therapy alone. In all 4 patients, successful treatment of the disease was established through either a follow-up panoramic radiograph or tissue biopsy, suggesting the efficacy of chemotherapy for non-Hogkin's lymphomas of the jaws.

Giant Cell Tumor of the Jaw

Giant cell tumors, although more prevalent in long bones, can present in the jaw. Branstetter and colleagues[29] found that giant cell tumors have high receptor activator of nuclear factor κ-B (RANK) ligand expression. Denosumab (Xgeva), a fully human monoclonal antibody, prevents RANK ligand-mediated formation and activation of multinucleated osteoclasts or giant cells by RANK-positive mononuclear preosteoclasts and macrophages, which in turn, suppresses bone destruction. Denosumab was then selected to treat 37 patients with recurrent or unresectable giant cell tumors of the bone. Locations of the tumor included the tibia, sacrum, femur, fibula, pubis, ulna, thoracic vertebrae, and radius. The denosumab dosage was 120 mg subcutaneously every 28 days, with additional doses on days 8 and 15. In on-study samples taken from 20 of 20 patients, decreases greater than or equal to 90% in giant tumor cells and in tumor stromal cells were observed, suggesting a promising role for denosumab in treating this type of tumor. Because this type of tumor can present itself in the jaws, although not in this study, Denusomab may show some efficacy in treatment based on this study's results.[30]

SUMMARY

Patients with oral cavity and maxillofacial cancers and postoperatively identified poor prognostic factors (eg, ECE, positive margins) benefit from the addition of adjuvant cisplatin-based chemotherapy to radiation therapy. In locally advanced tumors, a combination of cetuximab and radiation therapy is clearly more beneficial than radiation alone. Unfortunately, induction chemotherapy has not increased OS in patients with locally advanced head and neck tumors. In metastatic or inoperable recurrent disease, chemotherapy is used to prolong life and improve quality of life. In this setting, targeted therapy with cetuximab has been shown to be effective in combination with a platinum and 5-FU and the combination of cetuximab plus platinum and 5-FU is considered standard first-line therapy. Monotherapy with cetuximab or methotrexate could be considered for patients with poor PS. Many clinical trials investigating targeted therapies involving tyrosine kinase pathway and monoclonal antibodies are underway. Chemotherapy and targeted therapies play important roles in treating some rare oral and maxillofacial tumors, such as osteosarcomas, lymphomas, and giant cell tumors of the jaw.

ACKNOWLEDGMENTS

The authors acknowledge the help of Sunita Patterson, Scientific Editor, Department of Scientific Publications, The University of Texas MD Anderson Cancer Center.

REFERENCES

1. Siegel R, Naishadham D, Jemal A. Cancer statistics, 2013. CA Cancer J Clin 2013;63(1):11–30.

2. Siegel R, Naishadham D, Jemal A. Cancer statistics, 2013. CA Cancer J Clin 2012;62(1):10–29.
3. Shah J. Head and neck surgery. 2nd edition. London: Mosby-Wolfe; 1996.
4. Licitra L, Grandi C, Guzzo M, et al. Primary chemotherapy in resectable oral cavity squamous cell cancer: a randomized controlled trial. J Clin Oncol 2003; 21(2):327–33.
5. Zhong LP, Zhang CP, Ren GX, et al. Randomized phase III trial of induction chemotherapy with docetaxel, cisplatin, and fluorouracil followed by surgery versus up-front surgery in locally advanced resectable oral squamous cell carcinoma. J Clin Oncol 2013;31(6):744–51.
6. Hinerman RW, Mendenhall WM, Morris CG, et al. Postoperative irradiation for squamous cell carcinoma of the oral cavity: 35-year experience. Head Neck 2004;26(11):984–94.
7. Bernier J, Domenge C, Ozsahin M, et al. Postoperative irradiation with or without concomitant chemotherapy for locally advanced head and neck cancer. N Engl J Med 2004;350(19):1945–52.
8. Paccagnella A, Orlando A, Marchiori C, et al. Phase III trial of initial chemotherapy in stage III or IV head and neck cancers: a study by the Gruppo di Studio sui Tumori della Testa e del Collo. J Natl Cancer Inst 1994;86(4):265–72.
9. Posner MR, Hershock DM, Blajman CR, et al. Cisplatin and fluorouracil alone or with docetaxel in head and neck cancer. N Engl J Med 2007; 357(17):1705–15.
10. Vermorken JB, Remenar E, van Herpen C, et al. Cisplatin, fluorouracil, and docetaxel in unresectable head and neck cancer. N Engl J Med 2007;357(17): 1695–704.
11. Cohen E, Karrison T, Kocherginsky M. DeCIDE: a phase III randomized trial of docetaxel (D), cisplatin (P), 5-fluorouracil (F) (TPF) induction chemotherapy (IC) in patients with N2/N3 locally advanced squamous cell carcinoma of the head and neck (SCCHN). J Clin Oncol 2012;30(Suppl 15):5500.
12. Haddad R, O'Neill A, Rabinowits G, et al. Induction chemotherapy followed by concurrent chemoradiotherapy (sequential chemoradiotherapy) versus concurrent chemoradiotherapy alone in locally advanced head and neck cancer (PARADIGM): a randomised phase 3 trial. Lancet Oncol 2013;14: 257–64.
13. Bonner JA, Harari PM, Giralt J, et al. Radiotherapy plus cetuximab for locoregionally advanced head and neck cancer: 5-year survival data from a phase 3 randomised trial, and relation between cetuximab-induced rash and survival. Lancet Oncol 2010;11(1): 21–8.
14. Numico G, Franco P, Cristofano A, et al. Is the combination of Cetuximab with chemo-radiotherapy regimens worthwhile in the treatment of locally advanced head and neck cancer? A review of current evidence. Crit Rev Oncol Hematol 2013;85(2): 112–20.
15. Oken MM, Creech RH, Tormey DC, et al. Toxicity and response criteria of the Eastern Cooperative Oncology Group. Am J Clin Oncol 1982;5(6): 649–55.
16. Forastiere AA, Metch B, Schuller DE, et al. Randomized comparison of cisplatin plus fluorouracil and carboplatin plus fluorouracil versus methotrexate in advanced squamous-cell carcinoma of the head and neck: a Southwest Oncology Group study. J Clin Oncol 1992;10(8):1245–51.
17. Jacobs C, Lyman G, Velez-García E, et al. A phase III randomized study comparing cisplatin and fluorouracil as single agents and in combination for advanced squamous cell carcinoma of the head and neck. J Clin Oncol 1992;10(2):257–63.
18. Gibson MK, Li Y, Murphy B, et al. Randomized phase III evaluation of cisplatin plus fluorouracil versus cisplatin plus paclitaxel in advanced head and neck cancer (E1395): an intergroup trial of the Eastern Cooperative Oncology Group. J Clin Oncol 2005;23(15):3562–7.
19. Dassonville O, Formento JL, Francoual M, et al. Expression of epidermal growth factor receptor and survival in upper aerodigestive tract cancer. J Clin Oncol 1993;11(10):1873–8.
20. Vermorken JB, Mesia R, Rivera F, et al. Platinum-based chemotherapy plus cetuximab in head and neck cancer. N Engl J Med 2008;359(11):1116–27.
21. Vermorken JB, Trigo J, Hitt R, et al. Open-label, uncontrolled, multicenter phase II study to evaluate the efficacy and toxicity of cetuximab as a single agent in patients with recurrent and/or metastatic squamous cell carcinoma of the head and neck who failed to respond to platinum-based therapy. J Clin Oncol 2007;25(16):2171–7.
22. Kim E, Kies M, Glisson B. Final results of a phase II study of erlotinib, docetaxel and cisplatin in patients with recurrent/metastatic head and neck cancer. Paper presented at American Society of Clinical Oncology (ASCO) Annual Meeting. Chicago, IL.
23. Tabernero J. The role of VEGF and EGFR inhibition: implications for combining anti-VEGF and anti-EGFR agents. Mol Cancer Res 2007;5(3):203–20.
24. Viloria-Petit AM, Kerbel RS. Acquired resistance to EGFR inhibitors: mechanisms and prevention strategies. Int J Radiat Oncol Biol Phys 2004;58(3): 914–26.
25. Argiris A, Kotsakis AP, Hoang T, et al. Cetuximab and bevacizumab: preclinical data and phase II trial in recurrent or metastatic squamous cell carcinoma of the head and neck. Ann Oncol 2013;24(1):220–5.
26. DeAngelis AF, Spinou C, Tsui A, et al. Outcomes of patients with maxillofacial osteosarcoma: a review of 15 cases. J Oral Maxillofac Surg 2012;70(3):734–9.

27. Dhima M, Arce K, Moore EJ, et al. Novel oncologic, surgical, and prosthetic treatment of high-grade surface osteosarcoma, osteoblastic mandible type. J Oral Maxillofac Surg 2013;71(5):e224–31.

28. Pazoki A, Jansisyanont P, Ord RA. Primary non-Hodgkin's lymphoma of the jaws: report of 4 cases and review of the literature. J Oral Maxillofac Surg 2003;61(1):112–7.

29. Branstetter DG, Nelson SD, Manivel JC, et al. Denosumab induces tumor reduction and bone formation in patients with giant-cell tumor of bone. Clin Cancer Res 2012;18(16):4415–24.

30. Thomas D, Henshaw R, Skubitz K, et al. Denosumab in patients with giant-cell tumour of bone: an open-label, phase 2 study. Lancet Oncol 2010;11(3): 275–80.

Anti-Resorptive Osteonecrosis of the Jaws
Facts Forgotten, Questions Answered, Lessons Learned

Eric R. Carlson, DMD, MD*, Benjamin J. Schlott, DMD, MD

KEYWORDS

- Bisphosphonates • RANKL inhibitors • Metastatic cancer • Osteomyelitis • Osteonecrosis
- Resection

KEY POINTS

- Osteonecrosis of the jaws has been described in the literature for nearly 100 years in association with osteomyelitis, radiation therapy, with many medical conditions such as cancer and diabetes, and most recently in association with antiresorptive medications.
- Osteonecrosis of the jaws related to antiresorptive medications prescribed in the treatment of metastatic cancer and osteoporosis is poorly understood despite greater than 1 decade of recorded observations.
- Surgical resection of antiresorptive osteonecrosis of the jaws is highly curable and represents the preferred method of treatment of all stages of this disease provided that proper control of medical comorbidity has been accomplished.
- Untreated or conservatively managed asymptomatic early stage antiresorptive osteonecrosis of the jaws permits progression of the disease, thereby predisposing patients to the development of symptoms and ultimately necessitating resections of greater magnitude for advanced stage disease.
- Following resection, segmental defects related to antiresorptive osteonecrosis of the jaws are able to be successfully reconstructed with a variety of techniques.

If popular medicine gave the people wisdom as well as knowledge, it would be the best protection for scientific and well trained physicians.

—*Rudolf Virchow 1821–1902*

INTRODUCTION

Since 2003, health care providers have observed, managed, or been informed of the presence of osteonecrosis of the jaws in patients taking antiresorptive medications including bisphosphonate medications and human receptor activator for nuclear factor κ B ligand (RANKL) inhibitor medications.[1,2] In September 2003, Marx[3] published a letter to the editor in the *Journal of Oral and Maxillofacial Surgery* that reviewed 36 patients exposed to bisphosphonate medications with painful bone exposure in the jaws that were unresponsive to surgical or medical treatments.

Disclosure: Dr E.R. Carlson provides expert witness testimony for Hollingsworth LLP in re Aredia/Zometa litigation.

Department of Oral and Maxillofacial Surgery, University of Tennessee Medical Center, University of Tennessee Cancer Institute, 1930 Alcoa Highway, Knoxville, TN 37920, USA

* Corresponding author. Department of Oral and Maxillofacial Surgery, University of Tennessee Medical Center, University of Tennessee Cancer Institute, 1930 Alcoa Highway, Suite 335, Knoxville, TN 37920.

E-mail address: ecarlson@mc.utmck.edu

Oral Maxillofacial Surg Clin N Am 26 (2014) 171–191
http://dx.doi.org/10.1016/j.coms.2014.01.005
1042-3699/14/$ – see front matter © 2014 Elsevier Inc. All rights reserved.

Thirty-five of the patients were being treated for an underlying diagnosis of cancer and 1 patient was being treated for osteoporosis. Twenty-nine patients had osteonecrosis of the mandible, 5 had osteonecrosis of the maxilla, and 2 patients had osteonecrosis of the maxilla and mandible. Twenty-eight of the 36 patients had undergone extraction of a tooth. The author observed that the difficulty in treating the disease was that debridement could not be performed to uninvolved bone and may cause further exposure of bone. Prevention of the disease by avoiding tooth removal, controlling periodontal disease by nonsurgical means, avoiding the placement of dental implants, and using soft liners on dentures was most appropriate. It was also recommended that major debridement surgeries be avoided. The author reported that the diagnosis represented a previously unrecognized and unreported serious adverse effect and that caution should be exerted when prescribing bisphosphonate medications. In addition, the author indicated that, although no definite cause-and-effect relationship could be established between the bisphosphonate medications and the subsequent development of osteonecrosis of the jaws, these drugs were the direct factors in a multifactorial process leading to avascular necrosis of the jaws.

In 2003, Rosenberg and Ruggiero[4] reported 28 sites of osteonecrosis of the jaws in 26 patients who had cancer with metastatic bone disease and who had been exposed to bisphosphonate medications. Twenty-six sites were managed surgically and microscopic evaluation of these specimens did not identify metastatic disease. This study reported the possible association between bisphosphonate medications and the subsequent development of bisphosphonate-related osteonecrosis of the jaws (BRONJ) and represented a prelude to a publication by these investigators in 2004.[1] In this peer-reviewed publication, 72 sites of osteonecrosis were identified and managed in 63 patients, 56 of whom were treated with intravenous bisphosphonate medications and 7 of whom were treated with oral bisphosphonates. Among other issues, this report reviewed surgical therapy for this disease. Forty-five sequestrectomies, 4 marginal mandibular resections, 6 segmental mandibular resections, 5 partial maxillectomies, and 1 complete maxillectomy were performed. Two patients underwent observation of their disease. The investigators concluded that the management of patients with BRONJ was extremely difficult. Their surgical debridements were not completely effective in eradicating the necrotic bone. It was difficult in the senior author's experience to obtain a surgical margin with viable bleeding bone. They recommended, therefore, that surgical treatment be reserved only for those patients who were symptomatic, such as patients with a pathologic fracture associated with their osteonecrosis, in which case a segmental resection was indicated.

Numerous anecdotal case reports,[5,6] case series,[7–10] and position papers[11–13] were published after the first peer-reviewed article on BRONJ that served to provide information to health care providers regarding this disease process. The general consensus regarding treatment was that conservative, nonsurgical therapy was recommended to patients with asymptomatic disease, thereby reserving resection for advanced stage and symptomatic disease. In addition, beginning in 2010, reports were initially published in the literature that reviewed the presence of osteonecrosis of the jaws in patients exposed to denosumab, a RANKL monoclonal antibody.[2,14–16] These two forms of osteonecrosis of the jaws, those related to bisphosphonates and those related to denosumab, are now frequently and collectively referred to as antiresorptive osteonecrosis of the jaws (ARONJ).[17] In the 11 years since the original report on BRONJ, medical and dental professionals have continued to offer information on the pathogenesis and best form of treatment of osteonecrosis of the jaws associated with antiresorptive medications. This article reviews this information and draws on the clinical experience of the authors to remind the readership of the facts forgotten about osteonecrosis of the jaws. Questions regarding osteonecrosis of the jaws are answered and the lessons that have been learned are reviewed. Unless otherwise stated, osteonecrosis of the jaws related to bisphosphonate medications and RANKL inhibitors are collectively referred to as ARONJ.

OSTEONECROSIS OF THE JAWS IS SEEN IN PATIENTS WITHOUT CANCER WHO ARE NAIVE TO ANTIRESORPTIVE MEDICATIONS

Osteonecrosis of the jaws was not a new diagnosis when BRONJ was first described in 2003. In 1927, Blair and Brown[18] published a report of 15 cases of septic osteomyelitis of the bones of the skull and face in the *Annals of Surgery*. Three cases were located in the maxilla and 12 cases were located in the mandible. The investigators discussed 3 distinct clinical entities including the so-called ulcerated tooth, frank ostitis and necrosis of the dentigerous bones, and the spreading ostitis and necrosis that may accompany or follow purulent infection of the paranasal or para-aural sinuses. The investigators recommended the appropriate timing of the removal of all fragments of dead bone following control of the purulent infection. All 15 cases of osteomyelitis discussed in this article were accompanied by the development of osteonecrosis that was surgically removed. This treatment of the patients in this article did not involve antibiotic therapy because penicillin had yet to be discovered by Alexander Fleming in 1928. Nonetheless, the investigators treated some of their patients with osteomyelitis and osteonecrosis of the jaws with unspecified antisyphilitic treatment.

In 1938, Hankey[19] reported on the pathology and treatment of osteomyelitis and necrosis of the jaws. In particular, he indicated that osteomyelitis of the jaws occurred eighth in frequency of all of the bones in the body and 4 times more commonly in the mandible than the maxilla. Necrosis of the mandible was more common than that of the maxilla because the bone of the mandible is more dense and because the blood supply of the mandible is more easily obstructed.

In 1949, 4 articles were published that reviewed cases of osteomyelitis of the jaws in patients who were managed with surgical removal of necrotic bone, and some of whom also received antibiotic therapy.[20-23] These articles provided new observations related to osteomyelitis and osteonecrosis of the mandible, including the benefit of antibiotic therapy, the near-uniform presence of osteonecrosis in these cases, the occasional refractory nature of the treatment of osteomyelitis, and the preponderance of dental infections associated with the development of osteomyelitis and osteonecrosis of the jaws.

Contemporary writings on osteomyelitis and osteonecrosis of the jaws include a review of 141 cases of osteomyelitis by Adekeye and Cornah.[24] Of their 141 cases of osteomyelitis, 35 cases were located in the maxilla and 106 cases were located in the mandible. In descending order of prevalence, the possible causal factors for these cases of osteomyelitis included odontogenic infection, cancrum oris, tooth extraction, acute ulcerative gingivitis, fracture, and periodontal disease. Fracture, tooth extraction, and periodontal disease more likely resulted in osteomyelitis of the mandible, whereas acute ulcerative gingivitis and cancrum oris more likely resulted in osteomyelitis of the maxilla. The investigators reported that systemic medical compromise was of significance in the development of osteomyelitis in their patients, and comorbid medical conditions such as malnutrition, malaria, and anemia were more commonly associated with maxillary osteomyelitis than mandibular osteomyelitis. Only 4 patients (2.84%) had evidence of sickle cell anemia. The

investigators managed their cases of osteomyelitis with correction of malnutrition and treatment of other underlying medical comorbidities, culture-directed antibiotic therapy, and surgical therapy. Sequestrectomy, in particular, was performed in 26 and 61 cases of maxillary and mandibular osteomyelitis, respectively. Two cases of maxillary resection and 18 cases of mandibular resection were performed. The patients in this series were African and their presentations might therefore be considered to be atypical because of lack of access to health care, sanitation, and vaccination programs, with a resultant immunocompromised patient population.

In 2012, Khullar and colleagues[25] reported a case series of 60 cases of extreme osteonecrosis and osteomyelitis of the mandible and maxilla in a West African population. Fifty-four (90%) of these cases occurred in the mandible and 6 cases (10%) occurred in the maxilla. Exposed bone was noted in 31 cases; 30 extraorally and 1 intraorally. All patients were naive to bisphosphonate medications. All patients underwent surgical treatment of their osteomyelitis/osteonecrosis and 5 patients developed refractory disease that required additional surgery.

In 1991, Marx[26] reported specifically on chronic osteomyelitis of the jaws and offered a regimented treatment protocol. In particular, the presence of systemic disease that affects the immune response and wound healing is of causal significance in the development of osteomyelitis of the jaws. These diseases include diabetes, malnutrition, severe anemia, intravenous drug abuse, chronic alcoholism, and a variety of malignancies. In some of these diseases the immune system is suppressed to the point at which pus is no longer produced, such that a chronic nonsuppurative osteomyelitis occurs. The investigator's treatment protocol called for removal of the source of infection, debridement of necrotic tissue, obtaining a Gram stain and initiating empiric antibiotic therapy with the ultimate provision of culture-directed antibiotic therapy, and using hyperbaric oxygen therapy in refractory cases.

This historical perspective regarding osteomyelitis and osteonecrosis of the jaws serves as a reminder of some facts that may have been forgotten in the years since the original reports on this disease process. In particular, one lesson learned is that osteomyelitis of the jaws in compromised patients closely resembles osteonecrosis of the jaws in patients exposed to bisphosphonate medications. Both traditional osteomyelitis and ARONJ may be acute or chronic, suppurative or nonsuppurative, exacerbated by comorbid medical conditions, diagnosed in the maxilla and

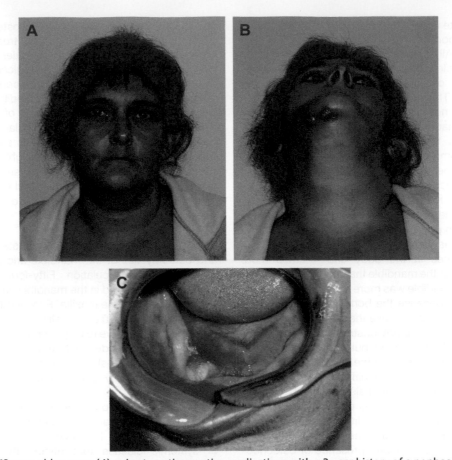

Fig. 1. A 42-year-old woman (*A*) naive to antiresorptive medications with a 2-year history of a nonhealing wound of the mandible and cutaneous fistulous tracts (*B*) following extraction of all of her remaining teeth in the mandible. She displayed exposed necrotic bone in the right mandible (*C*). Plain film (*D*) and computed tomography (CT) (*E*) radiographic evidence of sequestering bone of this region of the mandible was noted. A clinical and radiographic diagnosis of osteomyelitis with osteonecrosis of the mandible was established and the patient underwent a segmental resection of the mandible with excision of her fistulous tracts (*F*).

mandible, and ultimately defined by their presence of osteonecrosis (**Fig. 1**). Some cases of traditional osteomyelitis and BRONJ may become refractory to surgical therapy. Until BRONJ became considered a distinct pathologic entity in 2003, the presence of osteonecrosis in patients with osteomyelitis of the jaws was not specified in its nomenclature such that the existence of osteonecrosis in osteomyelitis had been forgotten, or at least underestimated. It has been forgotten that most cases of osteomyelitis of the jaws develop osteonecrosis given sufficient time to do so. As discussed elsewhere in this article, the lesson learned regarding ARONJ is that, like osteomyelitis, removal of osteonecrotic segments of the maxilla and mandible is essential for proper control of the disease, such that surgical therapy represents the most appropriate method of treatment of these two disease processes.

OSTEONECROSIS OF THE JAWS IS SEEN IN HIGHER INCIDENCES IN PATIENTS WITH CANCER

An analysis of the General Practice Research Database of 5.5 million patients in the United Kingdom indicated the incidence of osteonecrosis of all sites in the human body to be 4 times higher in patients with cancer than in the general population.[27] There are at least 3 explanations for this observation: the cancer's genetic blueprint; the host's medical comorbidity; and the treatment of the cancer, particularly related to chemotherapy. With regard to the cancer's genetic blueprint, it is known that cancers secrete a variety of cytokines that downregulate normal tissue homeostasis and upregulate their own blood supply and proliferation.[28] This observation becomes clinically apparent in cancer of the head and neck

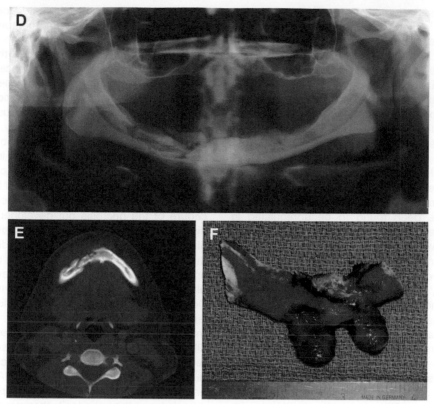

Fig. 1. (*continued*)

related to local and metastatic disease (**Fig. 2**). In general terms, osteolytic metastatic cancers disrupt the normal skeletal equilibrium such that bone formation and bone resorption are no longer coupled. The mechanism of metastatic breast cancer in bone resulting in osteonecrosis is well established and mediated through the binding of Fas-ligand (FasL) on breast cancer cells and Fas on osteoblasts.[29] It has been reported that normal breast epithelial cells express FasL and that this expression is upregulated in breast cancer tissue compared with normal breast and

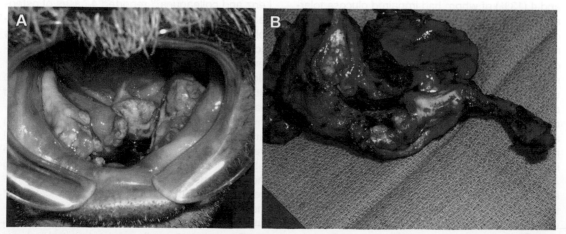

Fig. 2. A stage IV squamous cell carcinoma of the floor of mouth, mandibular gingiva, and mandible (*A*). Close examination identifies exposed necrotic bone, which becomes more apparent in the composite resection specimen (*B*).

benign breast tumor tissue.[30] Mastro and colleagues[31] suggested that the interaction of FasL on breast cancer cells and Fas on osteoblasts is a likely mechanism for breast cancer cell–mediated apoptosis of osteoblasts. Carlson and colleagues[32] speculated that this mechanism might explain the presence of osteonecrosis of the jaws in patients with metastatic breast cancer of the mandible and maxilla. The development of osteonecrosis in the mandible and maxilla related to a focus of metastatic disease can possibly also be explained by the expression of the matrix metalloproteinases (MMPs) by a variety of human cancers, including multiple myeloma.[32] The MMPs have been found to be upregulated in virtually every type of human cancer and are correlated with invasive and metastatic properties.[33] In addition, the upregulation of MMP-1, partial conversion of the pro–MMP-2 into its activated form, and production of MMP-7, MMP-8, MMP-9, and MMP-13 in multiple myeloma of the jaws may be related to the development of osteonecrosis in these sites.[32]

The patient's medical comorbidity is of great significance in the development of osteonecrosis of the jaws. Aside from the cancer and its inherent impairment of immune surveillance, the presence of diabetes mellitus, anemia, corticosteroid-dependent obstructive lung disease and rheumatologic disease, and other medical conditions serve to predispose the patient to the development of wound healing problems when undergoing a surgical procedure in the jaws or when patients sustain trauma from ill-fitting dentures. The effect of diabetes on the risk of osteonecrosis of the jaws has been perhaps the most widely discussed and studied comorbid medical condition. Khamaisi and colleagues[34] reported 31 patients with BRONJ, 14 of whom had type 2 diabetes (45%) and 4 (13%) of whom had impaired glucose tolerance. One patient had a history of gestational diabetes. Diabetes is generally associated with microvascular ischemia of bone, endothelial cell dysfunction, and decreased bone turnover and remodeling as well as induced apoptosis of osteoblasts and osteocytes. Favus[35] pointed out that diabetes may increase the risk of osteonecrosis of the jaws in the absence of microvascular disease and osteoclastic bone resorption of necrotic bone is impaired in experimental diabetes and bone infection.

The treatment of cancer frequently involves the administration of chemotherapy and many patients naive to bisphosphonate medications have developed osteonecrosis of the jaws in such settings.[36–40] In 1982, Schwartz[36] reported 2 cases of osteonecrosis of the jaws, 1 in the maxilla and

1 in the mandible, in patients treated for Hodgkin's disease with aggressive chemotherapy protocols, one of which included the administration of cyclophosphamide. Schwartz[36] indicated that the oral epithelium and marrow of the jaw bones are vulnerable to the destructive effects of chemotherapy protocols, and that osteomyelitis is more likely to occur in the compromised host because of inhibition of humoral and cellular immunity. Winer and colleagues[37] reported a case of osteonecrosis of the maxilla and palatal soft tissues in a patient treated with aggressive chemotherapy including cyclophosphamide for a diagnosis of lymphosarcoma. The patient underwent a debridement procedure of the necrosis but developed refractory disease that necessitated cessation of the cyclophosphamide. The investigators indicated that the necrosis was likely caused by this chemotherapeutic agent and an extensive review of cyclophosphamide was offered by the investigators. Developed in 1958, cyclophosphamide is an alkylating agent that is composed of a nitrogen mustard linked to a phosphoric acid derivative. Like other alkylating agents, cyclophosphamide interferes with rapidly dividing cells by cross-linking guanine bases, thereby preventing DNA replication and cell division. This ability to stop or disrupt mitosis forms the basis for its therapeutic and toxic effects. Certain tumor cell types, such as lymphocytes, are susceptible to alkylating agents. However, the drug's actions are not selective, such that rapidly dividing cells of the oral mucosa, the gastrointestinal tract, and hematopoietic tissue are particularly susceptible. Bagan and colleagues[38] reported 10 patients with osteonecrosis of the jaws in association with cancer chemotherapy. All of the patients received an intravenous bisphosphonate medication, whereas 8 of the patients also received cyclophosphamide. In 2005, Lenz and colleagues[39] reported 4 cases of osteonecrosis of the jaws in patients exposed to bisphosphonate medications. Two of the patients received Zometa and cyclophosphamide, 1 patient received ibandronate without cyclophosphamide, and 1 patient received cyclophosphamide with bisphosphonates. The investigators indicated that cancer chemotherapy can accelerate pathophysiologic events in the end arteries of the jaws within the bone marrow, and infarction of small branches of the nutrient artery can occur with the subsequent resorption of bony trabeculae. Sung and colleagues[40] similarly reported a case of osteonecrosis of the maxilla as a complication of chemotherapy in a patient naive to bisphosphonates. Their patient was treated with idarubicin and Cyparabine for a diagnosis of acute myelogenous leukemia. The patient developed necrotic

bone exposure in the maxilla that required debridement and primary closure of the oral mucosa. Hovi and colleagues[41] reported on opportunistic osteomyelitis in the jaws of children receiving immunosuppressive therapy who were naive to bisphosphonate medications. Three of the patients were diagnosed with acute lymphocytic leukemia and 1 patient was diagnosed with aplastic anemia. Three patients showed osteonecrosis of the mandible and 1 patient had osteonecrosis of the maxilla. Aside from their cancers, contributing factors to the development of osteonecrosis included 1 patient with type 1 diabetes mellitus, 2 patients receiving steroids, and 1 patient receiving cyclophosphamide. All patients underwent resection of their osteonecrosis and 2 patients required multiple surgeries because of the development of refractory osteonecrosis.

Osteonecrosis in patients with cancer is not a new phenomenon. Its presence in patients with lymphoma has been analyzed in particular.[42,43] Engel and colleagues[42] studied 17 patients with Hodgkin's lymphoma and 8 patients with non-Hodgkin's lymphoma who developed osteonecrosis of the femoral head or humeral head. All patients with Hodgkin's disease received combination chemotherapy with various cytotoxic agents and oral prednisone and all but 1 patient received radiotherapy with portals that included the eventually affected femoral or humeral head. The median interval from the termination of chemotherapy to the onset of osteonecrosis was 15 months, with a range of 0 to 54 months. Femoral osteonecrosis developed in 14 patients, of which 6 were unilateral and 8 were bilateral. Humeral osteonecrosis developed bilaterally in 2 patients and unilaterally in 1 patient. All patients with non-Hodgkin's lymphoma received various combined chemotherapy protocols that included intermittent oral prednisone. Five patients received moderate amounts of steroid-containing chemotherapy, whereas 3 patients were treated with high-dose steroid combination chemotherapy including cyclophosphamide. The median time interval from the diagnosis of the non-Hodgkin's lymphoma to the development of osteonecrosis was 39 months, with a range of 14 to 156 months. The investigators summarized their data of 25 cases of osteonecrosis in patients with lymphoma as representing 1.6% of the patients with Hodgkin's disease and 0.12% of the patients with non-Hodgkin's lymphoma treated between 1970 and 1979 at the Memorial Sloan Kettering Cancer Center. In 1985, Blijham and colleagues[43] described a case of osteonecrosis of the sternum and rib in a patient treated for Hodgkin's disease with

MOPP (Mustargen, Oncovin, Procarbazine, and Prednisone) chemotherapy and abdominopelvic radiation therapy. The osteonecrosis developed 23 months after the onset of treatment.

Perhaps the best known model of osteonecrosis of the jaws in patients with cancer not treated with radiation therapy is that of herpes zoster. This disease is an acute viral infection of the dorsal root ganglia of the spinal cord or the extramedullary cranial nerve ganglia. The condition is attributable to reactivation of latent varicella zoster virus in the dorsal root ganglia after an earlier outbreak of chicken pox. Alveolar bone necrosis in association with herpes zoster infection is a rare phenomenon but has been reported.[44,45] The exact mechanism by which herpes zoster causes jaw bone necrosis is uncertain. This uncertainty notwithstanding, it is possible that the neurotropic virus invades the sympathetic nerves that accompany the vasculature to the maxilla, thereby causing an intense vasoconstriction that leads to ischemia and necrosis in the maxillary bone, or possibly a vasculitis or endarteritis. Osteonecrosis associated with herpes zoster infection is more commonly observed in the maxilla than in the mandible.[46]

This historical perspective related to the development of osteonecrosis of the jaws in patients with cancer naive to bisphosphonate medications reveals numerous facts that may have been forgotten. The first is that osteonecrosis of the jaws does occur in this patient population and the literature is replete with examples describing such cases, similar to cases of osteonecrosis of the jaws occurring in patients exposed to bisphosphonate medications (**Fig. 3**). One of the common denominators is exposure to cytotoxic chemotherapy, particularly cyclophosphamide. In addition, patients develop osteonecrosis of other bones, including the femoral head, humeral head, and other bones when exposed to steroid-containing chemotherapeutic protocols for cancer, particularly lymphoma. It is therefore possible that the patient's cancer and the patient's cancer therapy are primarily responsible for the development of osteonecrosis of the jaws, with the bisphosphonate medication merely representing a cofactor.

TORI AND EXOSTOSES ARE AT-RISK STRUCTURES IN PATIENTS TAKING ANTIRESORPTIVE MEDICATIONS AND IN THOSE PATIENTS NAIVE TO ANTIRESORPTIVE MEDICATIONS

Mandibular tori, palatal tori, and buccal exostoses of the maxilla and mandible are nodular

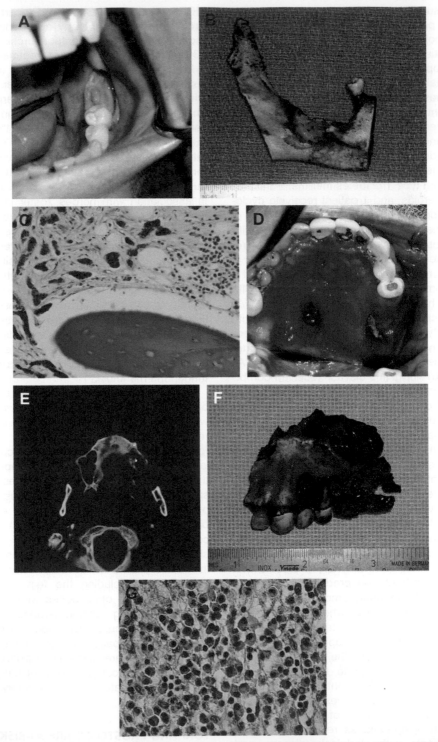

Fig. 3. Osteonecrosis of the left mandible (*A*) is noted in a patient who was treated with an aggressive chemotherapy protocol without antiresorptive medications for metastatic breast cancer. A segmental resection of the left mandible was performed (*B*), which showed microscopic signs of metastatic breast cancer in the background of osteonecrosis (*C*). Osteonecrosis is noted clinically (*D*) and radiographically (*E*) in the maxilla in a patient treated with bisphosphonate medications for a diagnosis of multiple myeloma. A partial maxillectomy was performed (*F*), which identified microscopic signs of osteonecrosis and multiple myeloma (*G*) ([C] hematoxylin and eosin, original magnification ×40; [G] hematoxylin and eosin, original magnification ×100).

protuberances of mature compact bone that represent anatomic variations of normal rather than pathologic conditions. Clinical experience and observations reveal that tori and exostoses of the maxilla and mandible can become exposed and necrotic in patients exposed to antiresorptive medications and in those patients naive to these medications (**Fig. 4**). Mandibular and palatal tori are typically asymptomatic and may show slow growth during the second and third decades of life.[47] The prevalence rate varies among studies and has been reported as high as 66% for palatal tori and 63.4% for mandibular tori. In the study of 1520 patients by Jainkittivong and colleagues,[47] 920 patients (60.5%) had palatal tori and 489 patients (32.2%) had mandibular tori. In their study

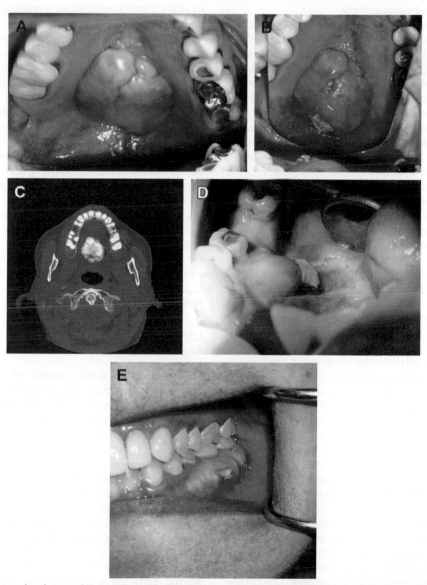

Fig. 4. A large palatal torus (*A*) in a 91-year-old patient naive to bisphosphonate medications. The significant magnitude of the torus precluded straightforward identification of osteonecrosis on its posterior surface, which only became apparent with indirect mirror evaluation (*B*). The result of the CT imaging is consistent with osteonecrosis of the palatal torus (*C*). Osteonecrosis may also be observed in association with mandibular tori, including in elderly patients who are bisphosphonate naive and who have large tori (*D*). Large lateral mandibular exostoses may also develop osteonecrosis (*E*) following surgical procedures, as occurred in this patient who underwent an apicoectomy on tooth #18.

of 960 patients, Jainkittivong and Langlais[48] identified 258 patients (26.9%) with exostoses, and indicated a greater than 5-fold incidence in the maxilla compared with the mandible. The prevalence of exostoses increased with age and they were significantly more common in men than in women. Sawair and colleagues[49] performed a cross-sectional study of 618 patients, 239 of whom (38.7%) had tori and exostoses. Mandibular tori were identified in 25.7% of their patients, and palatal tori and exostoses in 15.4% and 14.4% of their patients respectively.

The concept of osteonecrosis of jaw exostoses was first described by Peters and colleagues[50] in a study of 11 patients who had sequestra associated with ulceration of the lingual mucosa in the mylohyoid ridge region of the mandible. All of these cases developed in a spontaneous fashion and 7 patients underwent surgical removal, whereas 4 patients experienced spontaneous exfoliation of their sequestrum. The investigators offered a variety of local and systemic factors that might be implicated in this form of osteonecrosis. From a systemic perspective, only 1 patient carried a diagnosis of type 1 diabetes and was therefore predisposed to the development of wound healing problems. From a local perspective, the investigators identified the prominence of the mylohyoid ridge and its inherent injury-prone state. In addition, the deficient blood supply to this area of the mandible is thought to predispose this anatomic area to ulceration of the mucosa, superficial infection, reactive periostitis, and osteonecrosis.

Sonnier and Horning[51] reported 4 cases of spontaneous bony exposure of the jaws, with 3 of the cases occurring in the mandible and 1 case occurring in the maxilla. The report included 2 cases of osteonecrosis of mandibular tori, and 1 case each of osteonecrosis of the alveolus of the maxilla and a mandibular exostosis. The investigators suggested 5 possibilities to explain the cause of the exposed necrotic bone, including sharp projections from the tori causing chronic irritation; traumatic injury through sharp or hard foods, toothbrush injury, or oral habits; vascular constriction or embarrassment; excess occlusal forces or surgical trauma with thin overlying mucosa predisposed to dehiscence; and aphthous or vesiculobullous lesions.

In 2009, Almazrooa and Woo[52] provided a review of bisphosphonate and nonbisphosphonate-associated osteonecrosis of the jaws. The investigators conducted a literature search using PubMed to identify original research articles and case reports that described oral conditions and associated factors that result in sequestrum formation and bone exposure. In particular, the investigators reviewed idiopathic benign sequestration of the lingual plate of the mandible. This diagnosis consists of spontaneous sequestration of the lingual mandibular bone, usually in the area of the mylohyoid ridge, often in patients with no significant medical comorbidity. The investigators pointed out that thin mucosa overlies the mylohyoid ridge and that this tissue is more susceptible to subtle traumatic insults and ulceration even if patients do not report a history of trauma to this area. The attenuated blood supply to this area permits the development of osteonecrosis following dehiscence of the mucosa. Simple removal of the sequestrum permits complete healing without recurrence.

This literature review serves to affirm the lesson learned that osteonecrosis develops in tori and other exostoses of the jaws in patients exposed to and naive to bisphosphonate medications. The osteonecrosis seen in the mylohyoid ridge in patients exposed to bisphosphonate medications is like the osteonecrosis observed in the mylohyoid ridge in patients naive to bisphosphonates. These osteonecrotic sites are collectively seen in elderly compromised patients, including in those patients whose tori are large and subject to chronic trauma. As is the case with osteomyelitis with osteonecrosis, the nomenclature for a torus showing osteonecrosis has only included torus, without a specific reference to the presence of osteonecrosis. As such, the dearth of literature documenting this observation is likely representative of a lack of specific nomenclature rather than a lack of diagnosed cases.

UNTREATED OSTEONECROSIS OF THE JAWS PROGRESSES TO MORE ADVANCED STAGES

Following many initial reports of BRONJ and the recommendations of numerous investigators to provide conservative nonsurgical therapy, clinicians worldwide ultimately encountered patients with progressive disease. Although limited and uninfected early stage alveolar bone necrosis was initially diagnosed in many patients with BRONJ, nonsurgical therapy led to progression of disease with the development of suppurative infection, full-thickness involvement of the mandible, the development of maxillary sinusitis, and orocutaneous fistulae at unpredictable time points following initial diagnosis. It therefore seems logical that advanced disease developed from untreated and limited early stage disease and that successful resection of limited disease prevents the development of advanced stage disease. A comparison of serial clinical and radiographic examinations identifies the progression of the osteonecrosis and therefore supports this statement (**Fig. 5**). However, many investigators continue to recommend

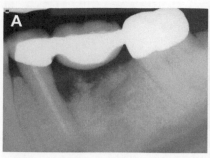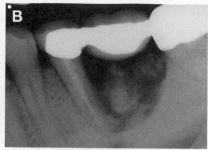

Fig. 5. A periapical radiograph of the left mandible (A) identifying the radiographic presentation of osteonecrosis in a 55-year-old man treated with bisphosphonates for multiple myeloma. A surgeon adopted conservative therapy for 9 months before referral for resection. The periapical radiograph obtained after 9 months of conservative therapy shows progression of the osteonecrosis (B).

nonsurgical therapy for stage 1 and 2 disease, suggesting the high likelihood that the exposed bone matures into a defined sequestrum that can be removed[53–55] such that surgical resection of BRONJ should be avoided.[56] However, clinical observation indicates that not only do these regions of necrotic bone most commonly not sequester but the magnitude of the osteonecrosis increases over time and asymptomatic patients become symptomatic. As discussed later, resection is successful BRONJ stage for BRONJ stage and therefore represents the preferable management strategy.

Watters and colleagues[56] presented their review of 154 patients diagnosed with BRONJ, 109 of whom had been treated with intravenous bisphosphonates. In particular, the investigators compared the stage and presentation of these patients at the first examination with the final follow-up examination to determine the clinical course. All patients were prescribed 0.12% chlorhexidine oral rinses and oral antibiotics when pain, swelling, or signs of infection existed. Surgical intervention was limited to marginal trimming of exposed bone and simple removal of bony sequestra. The clinical course was assessed as progressive, unchanged, partial resolution, and resolved. At variable and nonuniform final follow-up examinations, 26 patients (23.9%) were categorized as progressive, 42 patients (38.5%) were categorized as unchanged, 26 patients (23.9%) were categorized as partial resolution, and 6 patients (5.5%) were designated as resolved. The author's statistical analysis revealed that patients with a comorbid diagnosis of diabetes ($P = .05$), decayed/missing/filled teeth ($P = .02$), and pack-year tobacco history ($P = .03$) were more likely to have a progressive BRONJ outcome.

Clinical observation and objective data from the literature indicate that BRONJ progresses in its magnitude over time, although at an unpredictable rate, and that adopting a nonsurgical approach to BRONJ does not predictably result in sequestration of the exposed necrotic bone. Conservative therapy represents palliative rather than curative therapy in most cases of ARONJ. As discussed later, adopting a surgical approach to ARONJ results in a favorably high rate of resolution of osteonecrosis and avoids the development of refractory disease.

RESECTION REPRESENTS EFFECTIVE AND FIRST-LINE THERAPY FOR PATIENTS WITH OSTEONECROSIS OF THE JAWS

Osteonecrosis, by definition, represents dead bone. Dead tissue presents a surgical problem. The chronic presence of dead bone in the jaws, whether caused by osteoradionecrosis, by osteomyelitis, or of an unspecified cause, has always been approached with surgical debridement as part of a treatment algorithm. Surgical therapy remains the cornerstone of treating complex wounds of the human body, particularly when necrotic tissue is present.[57] In general terms, this therapy involves controlling bacterial burden; removing foreign bodies, debris, and necrotic tissue; and creating a sterile, well-vascularized, healthy wound bed amenable to primary closure or flap coverage. Antiresorptive osteonecrosis of the jaw represents a complex wound, in large part owing to the compromised nature of the patient. Based on all of these facts, ARONJ represents a surgical problem and surgery should be offered to most patients at the time of their diagnosis of osteonecrosis with the expressed intention of ending the progression of their osteonecrosis and curing it, while also maintaining their form and function (**Fig. 6**). Contrary to prior publications,[53–55] this approach is applied to all stages and locations of ARONJ in patients whose medical

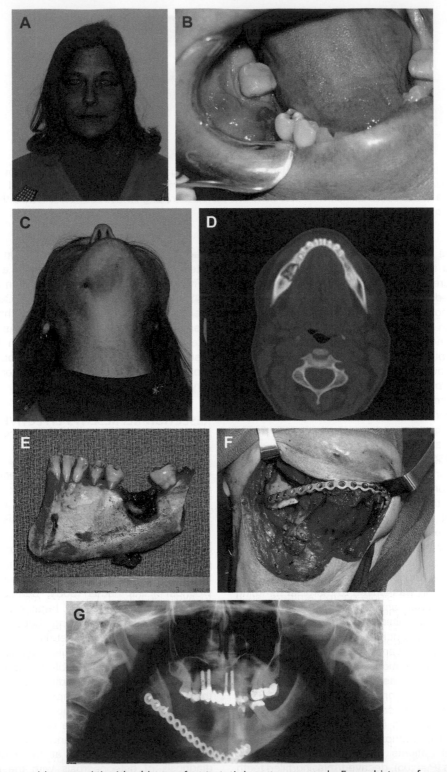

Fig. 6. A 51-year-old woman (*A*) with a history of metastatic breast cancer and a 5-year history of exposed bone in the right mandible (*B*). She had received intravenous bisphosphonate therapy for approximately 7 years related to metastatic breast cancer of the thoracic spine. She developed a fistulous tract in the neck approximately 6 months before referral (*C*). Radiographic imaging was consistent with a diagnosis of osteonecrosis of the right mandible (*D*). The patient underwent segmental resection of the right mandible (*E*) and immediate reconstruction with a bone plate (*F*, *G*). The patient healed without difficulty and no refractory disease developed.

comorbidity, metastatic disease burden, and social habits have been properly assessed and controlled, when possible.

Beginning in 2007, publications began to emerge that recommended surgical resection of BRONJ.[58–64] In 2007, Adornato and colleagues[58] reviewed the success of resection of 8 cases of BRONJ of the mandible that were refractory to conservative management and 4 cases of BRONJ of the maxilla. All patients had received intravenous bisphosphonate medications. All patients underwent a marginal resection of the mandible or an alveolectomy of the maxilla and all patients underwent the application of platelet-rich plasma to the resection site. Eight patients underwent a primary mucosal closure and the wounds of 4 patients were permitted to heal with secondary intention over a resorbable membrane. Ten of the 12 patients (83.3%) had maintained full mucosal coverage at an end point evaluation of 6 months. The investigators indicated that resection represented an effective treatment strategy for those cases of BRONJ that were refractory to conservative nonsurgical management.

In 2008, Abu-Id and colleagues[59] reported a multicenter retrospective study regarding BRONJ in 78 patients, including an assessment of the results of various forms of therapy. In 54 patients (69.2%) conservative surgical treatment including local debridement, decortication, and sequestrectomy was performed. These conservative measures were determined to be effective in only 38.5% of patients. Twenty-two patients underwent resection of their site of osteonecrosis and 19 patients (86.4%) were cured. Surgical resection had a better outcome than conservative therapy in this retrospective study. The investigators concluded that BRONJ should be approached with radical surgical resection to viable bone with a hermetic soft tissue closure.

In 2009, Carlson and Basile[60] reviewed 103 sites of BRONJ in 82 patients. Resection of 95 sites of osteonecrosis was performed in 74 patients. Sixty-six sites were resected in the mandible and 29 sites were resected in the maxilla. Fifty of the resected 95 sites were for stage I BRONJ, 32 sites were resected for stage II BRONJ, and 13 sites were resected for stage III BRONJ. Sixty-eight sites were resected in patients exposed to intravenous bisphosphonates, whereas 27 sites were resected in patients exposed to oral bisphosphonates. Of the 95 resected sites, 87 (91.6%) healed in an acceptable fashion, as noted by the maintenance of the oral mucosal closure over time and the presence of favorable radiographic remodeling. Of the 27 sites resected in patients taking oral bisphosphonate, 26 (96.3%) healed

acceptably. Of the 68 sites resected in patients given intravenous bisphosphonate, 61 (89.7%) healed acceptably. All 29 patients undergoing resection of the maxilla healed satisfactorily. Of the 8 sites of refractory osteonecrosis, 6 developed following a marginal resection of the mandible and 2 developed following segmental resection of the mandible.

In 2009, Stanton and Balasanian[61] reviewed a retrospective chart review of 51 patients with BRONJ, 33 of whom consented to surgical treatment. Four of the 33 patients were initially provided sequestrectomy under local anesthesia and 3 of these 4 patients healed in a satisfactory fashion. One patient required additional surgery. Twenty-five of the 33 patients had mandibular disease and 8 patients had maxillary disease. A total of 49 sites of BRONJ were surgically managed. The 33 studied patients underwent discontinuation of their bisphosphonate therapy at least 2 months before the planned surgical intervention. The bisphosphonate therapy was withheld for an additional 2 months after surgery. Debridement of all necrotic bone occurred in the operating room under general anesthesia for 29 of the patients. Antibiotics were administered during surgery, with levofloxacin being the antibiotic of choice of the investigators. Antibiotic therapy continued for at least 4 weeks after surgery. Hyperbaric oxygen therapy was not administered to the patients in this study. Twenty-eight of the 33 patients (85%) healed, as noted by complete mucosal coverage and elimination of pain with a follow-up period of 1 to 40 months (mean, 10.7 months). A total of 44 of the 49 sites (89.8%) were cured in these 33 patients. The investigators concluded that surgery was of benefit in the treatment of BRONJ and was highly successful in achieving a complete resolution of the process.

In 2010, Williamson[62] reported the results of surgical debridement of 40 patients with BRONJ who were followed after surgery for a period of 6 months to 4 years. The osteonecrosis occurred in the mandible in 25 patients and in the maxilla in 15 patients. Three cases had concurrent involvement of the maxilla and mandible. Patients were given either local or general anesthesia depending on the extent of the osteonecrosis. Williamson[62] performed debridement of the necrotic bone of the jaws, smoothing of sharp bony edges, and saucerization of any bony sockets. The author was often able to clearly identify surrounding viable bone, thereby assisting in the margin for the debridement. All of the 40 patients (100%) healed in a successful fashion with no wound breakdown occurring during follow-up.

In 2011, Wilde and colleagues[63] reported the role of surgical therapy in the management of intravenous BRONJ. Twenty-four patients with 33 sites of BRONJ, 19 sites located in the mandible and 14 sites located in the maxilla, were managed with a specific protocol that consisted of initial conservative therapy with oral peroxide rinses until surgery could be accomplished. Surgery consisted of resection of all infected necrotic bone to a margin of clinically apparent bleeding bone. Only 2 of the 19 sites of mandibular osteonecrosis necessitated a segmental resection. Bony margins were smoothed with a rotating bur followed by mobilization of a mucoperiosteal flap and a 2-layer closure. The investigators identified 29 of 33 resected sites (88%) of osteonecrosis to be resolved, as noted by the lack of exposed bone, no mucosal defect, no fistulae, and the absence of swelling and pain. The investigators concluded their study by stating that patients with BRONJ may benefit from surgical treatment, especially those patients who still have a reasonable life expectancy and high quality of life.

The previously cited articles examined the efficacy of resection or surgical debridement of BRONJ with curative intent. In 2008, Wutzl and colleagues[64] reported the results of intentional incomplete sequestrectomy and debridement of osteonecrotic bone in 58 patients who had been treated with bisphosphonate medications. When sequestrectomy and decortication with local soft tissue closure under general anesthesia was performed, the investigators did not attempt to establish viable bone margins by removing all of the necrotic bone. Twenty-four of 41 patients (55.8%) who underwent surgery and who were available for follow-up had an intact mucosa noted at 6 months after surgery. In 2012, Graziani and colleagues[65] performed a retrospective cohort multicenter study of 347 patients with BRONJ. In particular, the investigators determined the success of debridement versus resection of the sites of osteonecrosis. Of the 347 patients, 227 underwent local debridement and 120 underwent resection. Following surgical debridement, 49% of cases showed improvement, with no improvement in 33% of cases and worsening in the remaining 16%. Resection resulted in a statistically significant difference ($P = .002$) with improvement seen in 68% of cases, no improvement in 27% of cases, and worsening in 5% of cases. The investigators concluded that resection achieved a higher rate of clinical success compared with local debridement, and that a multivariate analysis indicated that maxillary location, resective surgery, and the

absence of a corticosteroid treatment regimen were associated with a positive outcome.

Clinical experience and this review of the literature show that resection is an effective method of cure for patients with BRONJ. This approach should be applied to patients with all stages of ARONJ, including stage I disease.[66] This notwithstanding, it is paramount to provide proper control of the patient's comorbid medical conditions, including effective glycemic control in diabetic patients, correction of anemia, and an assessment of the burden of metastatic disease with proper treatment before executing resection of ARONJ. Another lesson learned is that physiologically compromised patients, such as those with an increasing burden of distant metastatic disease, may not respond favorably to resection of their osteonecrotic jaws, and may occasionally develop refractory disease.

MANDIBULAR SEGMENTAL DEFECTS CAN BE RECONSTRUCTED IN PATIENTS EXPOSED TO BISPHOSPHONATE MEDICATIONS

The need for reconstruction of segmental defects of the mandible related to ARONJ has become more common over the past decade as surgeons have become more accepting of the appropriateness of resection of this disease process. In addition, large segmental resections have become required since many patients with BRONJ were conservatively managed because of earlier concern for the efficacy of resection, thereby promoting the progression of early stage disease to more advanced stage disease. As patients with cancer and BRONJ have been cured of their osteonecrosis, and as these patients treated with bisphosphonate medications have experienced longer palliation of their underlying malignant processes, the appropriateness of definitive reconstruction of segmental defects of the mandible has been realized. To this end, several methods of mandibular reconstruction are worthy of discussion.

Immediate reconstruction of segmental defects created by ARONJ resections is accomplished with reconstruction bone plates,[67] free microvascular flaps,[68] and recombinant bone morphogenetic protein-2 (rhBMP-2).[69] Marx[67] pointed out that reconstruction bone plates should be placed with precision with the intent of long-term use in patients with cancer because of the likelihood that these patients will not become candidates for definitive bone graft reconstruction. In particular, he recommended the placement of 4 to 5 bicortical screws in each mandibular segment. This exercise is typically uncomplicated because of the ability to anatomically and precisely place the bone plate on the unresected mandible, thereby preserving the patient's occlusion and also avoiding the need for maxillomandibular fixation during the placement of the bone plate. Clinical experience shows that not only is the identification of viable bone able to be realized in these resections but the remaining viable bone, complexed with bisphosphonate medications, tolerates bicortical screw placement and maintains their integrity for long periods of time without becoming necrotic.

It has been the authors' experience and that of others that autogenous particulate bone graft reconstruction of ARONJ-related segmental defects of the mandible is highly successful, including that performed in patients with cancer (**Fig. 7**). Although Marx[67] originally recommended such reconstructions in patients with prostate and metastatic breast cancer, he recommended against this type of reconstruction in patients with multiple myeloma because of the potential for bone marrow involvement by this malignant diagnosis. This notwithstanding, a thorough preoperative assessment of patients with multiple myeloma with serum protein electrophoresis and plain films of the ilium may permit the selection of patients without involvement of their donor site of the ilium. Along with intraoperative submission of iliac cancellous bone for permanent section histopathologic assessment of the presence of multiple myeloma, this often results in the ability to reconstruct these patients with tumor-free cancellous bone. The use of plain films, bone scans, and positron emission tomography scans should be obtained before surgery in patients with metastatic prostate and breast cancer with ARONJ-related segmental defects of the

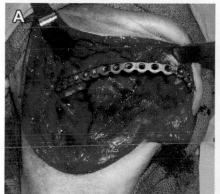
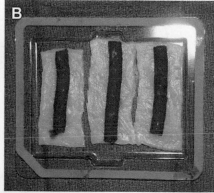
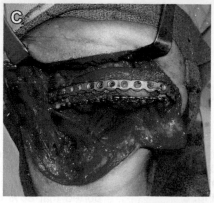

Fig. 7. The patient whose resection was shown in **Fig. 6** was prepared for bone graft reconstruction of her right mandibular segmental defect. A strictly transcutaneous approach was followed and the scarred defect was developed (*A*). A graft system consisting of autogenous cancellous bone combined with rhBMP-2 in an absorbable collagen sponge was created (*B*). The graft was placed in the defect (*C*) and its placement is noted radiographically immediately after surgery (*D*). Consolidation and remodeling of the graft was noted at 4 months after surgery (*E*) such that bone remodeling suppression was not at work in this patient. The patient was planned for navigational implant placement (*F, G*). She showed excellent clinical (*H, I*) and radiographic (*J*) healing, as noted at 2 years after surgery, and she subsequently underwent dental rehabilitation (*K, L*). The prosthodontics were provided by Dr Steven LoCascio, Knoxville, Tennessee.

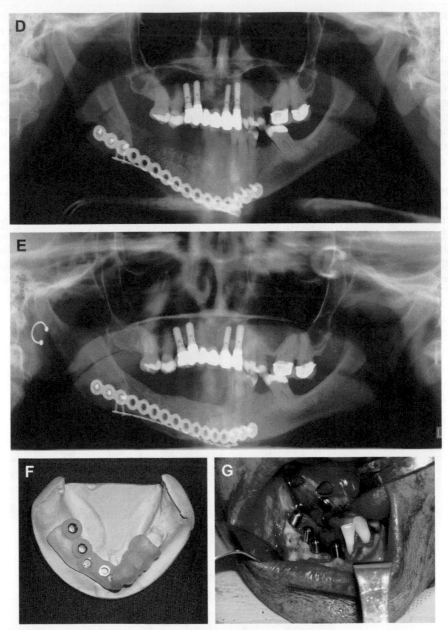

Fig. 7. (*continued*)

mandible in preparation for autogenous bone graft reconstruction so as to provide reasonable certainty as to whether a tumor-free donor site exists for such reconstructions (**Fig. 8**).

TEETH MAY BE EXTRACTED IN PATIENTS EXPOSED TO BISPHOSPHONATE MEDICATIONS WITHOUT THE SUBSEQUENT DEVELOPMENT OF OSTEONECROSIS

Initial reports[1,70] and subsequent reports[71–73] identified tooth extraction as a major risk factor

for the development of osteonecrosis of the jaws in patients exposed to bisphosphonate medications. Ruggiero and colleagues[1] originally reported that 86% of their 63 patients developed BRONJ following tooth extraction. Ficarra and colleagues'[70] series of 9 patients uniformly developed osteonecrosis of the jaws following tooth extraction. In a series of 22 patients with BRONJ, Badros and colleagues[71] determined that the predicted risk of developing osteonecrosis was 9 times greater following extraction of a tooth. Vahtsevanos and colleagues[72] calculated the

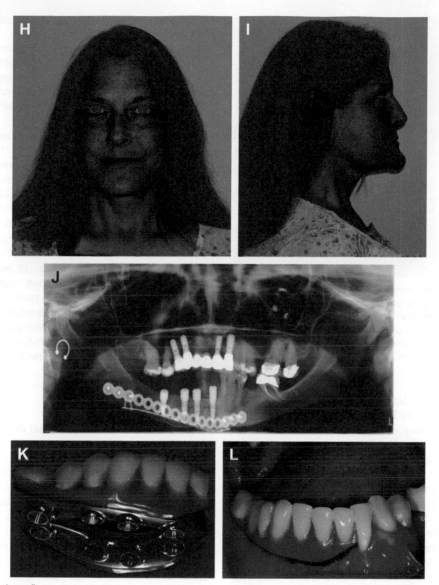

Fig. 7. (*continued*)

relative risk for development of osteonecrosis of the jaws to be 18 times higher in patients who underwent dental extractions. When this risk was approximated via regression modeling and after adjusting for a series of possible confounders, it was determined to be as high as 33-fold. These publications and others resulted in what could be described as panic on the part of dental professionals caring for bisphosphonate-exposed patients.[74] However, the question remained, could patients undergo dental extractions without developing osteonecrosis? Beginning in 2010, reports were published that showed the safety of tooth extraction in bisphosphonate-exposed patients.[75–77] Lodi and colleagues[75] prospectively

reported on 38 extractions in 23 patients who had been treated with intravenous bisphosphonates for a mean of 17.5 months. A protocol of preoperative and postoperative antibiotics was observed for all patients. The investigators meticulously curetted the extraction sockets and provided primary mucosal coverage over the extraction sockets. No cases of osteonecrosis followed tooth extraction in their series. The investigators concluded that an absolute contraindication to tooth extraction in patients taking intravenous bisphosphonates does not exist. Periodontal and dental abscesses associated with hopeless teeth in this patient cohort represent a risk factor for BRONJ that is similar to

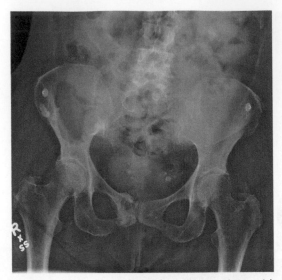

Fig. 8. A plain film of the hip in a patient with metastatic disease of the right ilium. Obtaining plain films of potential donor sites in patients with segmental defects of the mandible related to ARONJ represents a minimum parameter before committing to bone harvest at that donor site for mandibular reconstruction.

that of an extraction because both conditions increase the risk of BRONJ 7-fold.[11] In 2011, Scoletta and colleagues[76] prospectively reported on 220 extractions in 64 consecutive patients exposed to intravenous bisphosphonate therapy. Preoperative antibiotics were given to all patients. All extraction sockets were filled with autologous plasma rich in growth factors (PRGF) and a primary closure of the extraction sites was accomplished with a vestibular soft tissue flap. Five patients developed BRONJ in 5 extraction sockets (2.27%). The investigators concluded that their prospective study showed that their treatment protocol provided the safe removal of teeth and reduced the frequency of postoperative BRONJ development. In 2013, Scoletta and colleagues[77] reported on a more rapid protocol for tooth extraction in intravenous bisphosphonate–exposed patients. Sixty-three patients underwent 202 tooth extractions after initiating oral antibiotic therapy on the evening before surgery. The investigators removed the teeth and placed autologous PRGF in the extraction sites. They modified their technique for mucosal closure by only providing simple cross-suturing and incomplete mucosal closure for maintenance and stability of the PRGF rather than an elaborate soft tissue flap that ensured full mucosal closure. BRONJ was noted to develop in 2 extraction sockets (0.99%) in 1 patient after surgery. In addition, Mavrokokki and colleagues[78] specifically assessed the risk

of osteonecrosis of the jaws in patients exposed to oral bisphosphonate medications. The risk of osteonecrosis in osteoporotic patients taking alendronate was 1 in 2260 to 1 in 8470 patients (0.01%–0.04%). If extractions were performed in these patients, the calculated frequency was 1 in 296 to 1 in 1130 cases (0.09%–0.34%); still an infrequent event.

The prior studies show that teeth can be safely removed in patients exposed to intravenous and oral bisphosphonate medications without a significant risk for the postoperative development of BRONJ. As such, surgeons should proceed with tooth extraction in this patient cohort with the recognition that the incidence of osteonecrosis is low in these patients such that forced eruption of teeth[79,80] is not necessary in an effort to avoid the development of osteonecrosis. In addition, the increased risk of spontaneous osteonecrosis development in patients with periodontitis[81] requires that hopeless teeth be removed in patients exposed to bisphosphonate medications. Avoiding the extraction of such teeth for fear of developing trauma-induced osteonecrosis may be counterproductive.

SUMMARY

In the 11 years since its original description, the diagnosis, pathophysiology, prevention, and most effective treatment of BRONJ have been debated and disputed such that opinions have occasionally replaced facts and observational dogma has occasionally substituted for evidence-based recommendations. Although the pathophysiology and causation of ARONJ remain controversial, surgical treatment is approaching consensus such that patients are able to be treated with predictable resection and reconstruction.

REFERENCES

1. Ruggiero S, Mehrotra B, Rosenberg T. Osteonecrosis of the jaws associated with the use of bisphosphonates: a review of 63 cases. J Oral Maxillofac Surg 2004;62:527–34.
2. Aghaloo T, Felsenfeld A, Tetradis S. Osteonecrosis of the jaw in a patient on denosumab. J Oral Maxillofac Surg 2010;68:959–63.
3. Marx RE. Pamidronate (Aredia) and zoledronate (Zometa) induced avascular necrosis of the jaws: a growing epidemic. J Oral Maxillofac Surg 2003; 61:1115–8.
4. Rosenberg T, Ruggiero S. Osteonecrosis of the jaws associated with the use of bisphosphonates. J Oral Maxillofac Surg 2003;61(Suppl 1):60.

5. Levin L, Laviv A, Schwartz-Arad D. Denture-related osteonecrosis of the maxilla associated with oral bisphosphonate treatment. J Am Dent Assoc 2007; 138:1218–20.

6. Dodson RB, Raje NS, Caruso PA, et al. Case 9-2008: a 65-year old woman with a nonhealing ulcer of the jaw. N Engl J Med 2008;358:1283–91.

7. Dimopoulos MA, Kastritis E, Anagnostopoulos A, et al. Osteonecrosis of the jaw in patients with multiple myeloma treated with bisphosphonates: evidence of increased risk after treatment with zoledronic acid. Haematologica 2006;91:970–3.

8. Bamias A, Kastritis E, Bamia C, et al. Osteonecrosis of the jaw in cancer after treatment with bisphosphonates: incidence and risk factors. J Clin Oncol 2005;23:8580–7.

9. Boonyapakorn T, Schirmer I, Reichart PA, et al. Bisphosphonate-induced osteonecrosis of the jaws: prospective study of 80 patients with multiple myeloma and other malignancies. Oral Oncol 2008;44(9):857–69.

10. Migliorati CA, Schubert MM, Peterson DE, et al. Bisphosphonate-associated osteonecrosis of mandibular and maxillary bone. An emerging oral complication of supportive cancer therapy. Cancer 2005;104:83–93.

11. Advisory Task Force on Bisphosphonate-related Osteonecrosis of the Jaws, American Association of Oral and Maxillofacial Surgeons. American Association of Oral and Maxillofacial Surgeons position paper on bisphosphonate-related osteonecrosis of the jaws. J Oral Maxillofac Surg 2007;65: 369–76.

12. Migliorati CA, Casiglia J, Epstein J. Managing the care of patients with bisphosphonate-related osteonecrosis. An American Academy of Oral Medicine position paper. J Am Dent Assoc 2005;136: 1658–68.

13. Woo SB, Hellstein JW, Kalmar JR. Systematic review: bisphosphonates and osteonecrosis of the jaws. Ann Intern Med 2006;144:753–61.

14. Stopeck AT, Lipton A, Body JJ, et al. Denosumab compared with zoledronic acid for the treatment of bone metastases in patients with advanced breast cancer: a randomized, double-blind study. J Clin Oncol 2010;28:5132–9.

15. Diz P, Lopez-Cedrun JL, Arenaz J, et al. Denosumab-related osteonecrosis of the jaw. J Am Dent Assoc 2012;143:981–4.

16. Taylor K, Middlefell L, Mizen K. Osteonecrosis of the jaws induced by anti-RANK ligand therapy. Br J Oral Maxillofac Surg 2010;48:221–3.

17. Hellstein JW, Adler RA, Edwards B, et al. Managing the care of patients receiving anti-resorptive therapy for prevention and treatment of osteoporosis: executive summary of recommendations from the American Dental Association Council on Scientific Affairs. J Am Dent Assoc 2011;142: 1243–51.

18. Blair VP, Brown JB. Septic osteomyelitis of the bones of the skull and face. Ann Surg 1927;85:1–26.

19. Hankey GT. Osteomyelitis (necrosis) of the jaws – its pathology and treatment. Br Dent J 1938;65: 550–9.

20. Parker DB. Osteomyelitis of the mandible: report of case. J Oral Surg 1949;7:69–71.

21. Karpawich AJ. Chemotherapy of osteomyelitis of the mandible: report of case. J Oral Surg 1949;7: 76–8.

22. Wass SH. Osteomyelitis of the mandible. Ann R Coll Surg Engl 1949;4:48–57.

23. England LC, Golan HP. Two cases of acute osteomyelitis of the mandible. Oral Surg Oral Med Oral Pathol 1949;2:1522–9.

24. Adekeye EO, Cornah J. Osteomyelitis of the jaws: a review of 141 cases. Br J Oral Maxillofac Surg 1985;23:24–35.

25. Khullar SM, Tvedt D, Chapman K, et al. Sixty cases of extreme osteonecrosis and osteomyelitis of the mandible and maxilla in a West African population. Int J Oral Maxillofac Surg 2012;41:978–85.

26. Marx RE. Chronic osteomyelitis of the jaws. Oral Maxillofac Surg Clin North Am 1991;3:367–81.

27. Tarassoff P, Csermak K. Avascular necrosis of the jaws: risk factors in metastatic cancer patients. J Oral Maxillofac Surg 2003;61:1238–9.

28. Marx RE. Oral and intravenous bisphosphonate-induced osteonecrosis of the jaws: history, etiology, prevention and treatment. 2nd edition. Chicago: Quintessence Publishing; 2011. p. 45–70.

29. Fromigue O, Kheddoumi N, Lomri A, et al. Breast cancer cells release factors that induce apoptosis in human bone marrow stromal cells. J Bone Miner Res 2001;16:1600–10.

30. Mullauer L, Mosberger I, Gusch M, et al. Fas ligand is expressed in normal breast epithelial cells and is frequently upregulated in breast cancer. J Pathol 2000;190:20–30.

31. Mastro AM, Gay CV, Welch DR, et al. Breast cancer cells induce osteoblast apoptosis: a possible contributor to bone degradation. J Cell Biochem 2004;91:265–76.

32. Carlson ER, Fleisher K, Ruggiero SL. Metastatic cancer identified in osteonecrosis specimens of the jaws in patients receiving intravenous bisphosphonates medications. J Oral Maxillofac Surg 2013;71(12):2077–86.

33. Coussens I, Fingleton B, Matrisian I. Matrix metalloproteinase inhibitors and cancer: trials and tribulations. Science 2002;295:2387–92.

34. Khamaisi M, Regev E, Yarom N, et al. Possible association between diabetes and bisphosphonates-related jaw osteonecrosis. J Clin Endocrinol Metab 2007;92:1172–5.

35. Favus MJ. Diabetes and the risk of osteonecrosis of the jaw. J Clin Endocrinol Metab 2007;92:817–8.

36. Schwartz HC. Osteonecrosis of the jaws: a complication of cancer chemotherapy. Head Neck Surg 1982;4:251–3.

37. Winer HJ, McMahon RE, Olson RE. Palatal necrosis secondary to cytoxin therapy: report of case. J Am Dent Assoc 1972;84:862–6.

38. Bagan JV, Murillo J, Jimenez Y, et al. Avascular jaw osteonecrosis in association with cancer chemotherapy: series of 10 cases. J Oral Pathol Med 2005;34:120–3.

39. Lenz J-H, Steiner-Krammer B, Schmidt W, et al. Does avascular necrosis of the jaws in cancer patients only occur following treatment with bisphosphonates? J Craniomaxillofac Surg 2005;33:395–403.

40. Sung EC, Chan SM, Sakurai K, et al. Osteonecrosis of the maxilla as a complication to chemotherapy: a case report. Spec Care Dentist 2002;22:142–6.

41. Hovi L, Saarinen UM, Donner U, et al. Opportunistic osteomyelitis in the jaws of children on immunosuppressive chemotherapy. J Pediatr Hematol Oncol 1996;18:90–4.

42. Engel IA, Straus DJ, Lacher M, et al. Osteonecrosis in patients with malignant lymphoma: a review of twenty-five cases. Cancer 1981;48:1245–50.

43. Blijham GH, Vermeulen A, Mendes de Leon DE. Osteonecrosis of sternum and rib in a patient treated for Hodgkin's disease. Cancer 1985;56:2292–4.

44. Owotade FJ, Ugboko VI, Kolude B. Herpes zoster infection of the maxilla: case report. J Oral Maxillofac Surg 1999;57:1249–51.

45. Pogrel MA, Miller CE. A case of maxillary necrosis. J Oral Maxillofac Surg 2003;61:489–93.

46. Muto T, Tsuchiya H, Sato K, et al. Tooth exfoliation and necrosis of the mandible – a rare complication following trigeminal herpes zoster: report of a case. J Oral Maxillofac Surg 1990;48:1000–3.

47. Jainkittivong A, Apinhasmit W, Swasdison S. Prevalence and clinical characteristics of oral tori in 1,520 Chulalongkorn University Dental School patients. Surg Radiol Anat 2007;29:125–31.

48. Jainkittivong A, Langlais RP. Buccal and palatal exostoses: prevalence and concurrence with tori. Oral Surg Oral Med Oral Pathol Oral Radiol Endod 2000;90:48–53.

49. Sawair FA, Shayyab MH, Al-Rababah MA, et al. Prevalence and clinical characteristics of tori and jaw exostoses in a teaching hospital in Jordan. Saudi Med J 2009;30(12):1557–62.

50. Peters E, Lovas GL, Wysocki GP. Lingual mandibular sequestration and ulceration. Oral Surg Oral Med Oral Pathol 1993;75:739–43.

51. Sonnier KE, Horning GM. Spontaneous bony exposure: a report of 4 cases of idiopathic exposure and sequestration of alveolar bone. J Periodontol 1997;68:758–62.

52. Almazrooa SA, Woo SB. Bisphosphonate and nonbisphosphonate-associated osteonecrosis of the jaw. A review. J Am Dent Assoc 2009;140:864–75.

53. Ruggiero SL. Emerging concepts in the management and treatment of osteonecrosis of the jaw. Oral Maxillofac Surg Clin North Am 2013;25:11–20.

54. Moretti F, Pelliccioni GA, Montebugnoli L, et al. A prospective clinical trial for assessing the efficacy of a minimally invasive protocol in patients with bisphosphonates-associated osteonecrosis of the jaws. Oral Surg Oral Med Oral Pathol Oral Radiol Endod 2011;112:777–82.

55. Marx RE. Oral and intravenous bisphosphonate-induced osteonecrosis of the jaws. History, etiology, prevention, and treatment. Chicago: Quintessence Publishing; 2011. p. 60.

56. Watters AL, Hansen HJ, Williams T, et al. Intravenous bisphosphonate-related osteonecrosis of the jaw: long-term follow-up of 109 patients. Oral Surg Oral Med Oral Pathol Oral Radiol Endod 2013;115:192–200.

57. Park H, Copeland C, Henry S, et al. Complex wounds and their management. Surg Clin North Am 2010;90:1181–94.

58. Adornato MC, Morcos I, Rozanski J. The treatment of bisphosphonate-associated osteonecrosis of the jaws with bone resection and autologous platelet-derived growth factors. J Am Dent Assoc 2007;138:971–7.

59. Abu-Id MH, Warnke PH, Gottschalk J, et al. "Bisphossy jaws" – high and low risk factors for bisphosphonate-induced osteonecrosis of the jaw. J Craniomaxillofac Surg 2008;36:95–103.

60. Carlson ER, Basile JD. The role of surgical resection in the management of bisphosphonate related osteonecrosis of the jaws. J Oral Maxillofac Surg 2009;67(Suppl 1):85–95.

61. Stanton DC, Balasanian E. Outcome of surgical management of bisphosphonate-related osteonecrosis of the jaws: review of 33 surgical cases. J Oral Maxillofac Surg 2009;67(5):943–50.

62. Williamson RA. Surgical management of bisphosphonate induced osteonecrosis of the jaws. Int J Oral Maxillofac Surg 2010;39:251–5.

63. Wilde F, Heufelder M, Winter K, et al. The role of surgical therapy in the management of intravenous bisphosphonate-related osteonecrosis of the jaw. Oral Surg Oral Med Oral Pathol Oral Radiol Endod 2011;111:153–63.

64. Wutzl A, Biedermann E, Wanschitz F, et al. Treatment results of bisphosphonate-related osteonecrosis of the jaws. Head Neck 2008;30:1224–30.

65. Graziani F, Vescovi P, Campisi G, et al. Resective surgical approach shows a high performance

in the management of advanced cases of bisphosphonate-related osteonecrosis of the jaws: a retrospective survey of 347 cases. J Oral Maxillofac Surg 2012;70:2501–7.

66. Kyrgidis A, Koloutsos G, Vahtsevanos K. Treatment protocols of bisphosphonate-related osteonecrosis of the jaws [letter to the editor]. Head Neck 2009; 31:1112–3.

67. Marx RE. Reconstruction of defects caused by bisphosphonate-induced osteonecrosis of the jaws. J Oral Maxillofac Surg 2009;67(Suppl 1):107–19.

68. Engroff SL, Kim DD. Treating bisphosphonate osteonecrosis of the jaws: is there a role for resection and vascularized reconstruction? J Oral Maxillofac Surg 2007;65:2374–85.

69. Herford AS, Boyne PJ. Reconstruction of mandibular continuity defects with bone morphogenetic protein-2 (rhBMP-2). J Oral Maxillofac Surg 2008; 66:616–24.

70. Ficarra G, Beninati F, Rubino I, et al. Osteonecrosis of the jaws in periodontal patients with a history of bisphosphonate therapy. J Clin Periodontol 2005; 32:1123–8.

71. Badros A, Weikel D, Salama A, et al. Osteonecrosis of the jaw in multiple myeloma patients: clinical features and risk factors. J Clin Oncol 2006;24:945–52.

72. Vahtsevanos K, Kyrgidis A, Verrou E, et al. Longitudinal cohort study of risk factors in cancer patients of bisphosphonate-related osteonecrosis of the jaw. J Clin Oncol 2009;27:5356–62.

73. Kyrgidis A, Vahtsevanos K, Koloutsos G, et al. Bisphosphonate-related osteonecrosis of the jaws: a case-control study of risk factors in breast cancer patients. J Clin Oncol 2008;26:4634–8.

74. Carlson ER. Bisphosphonate related osteonecrosis of the jaws. An old disease with a new drug? Cranio 2010;28:1–2.

75. Lodi G, Sardella A, Salis A. Tooth extraction in patients taking intravenous bisphosphonates: a preventive protocol and case series. J Oral Maxillofac Surg 2010;68:107–10.

76. Scoletta M, Arduino PG, Pol R. Initial experience on the outcome of teeth extractions in intravenous bisphosphonate-treated patients: a cautionary report. J Oral Maxillofac Surg 2011;69:456–62.

77. Scoletta M, Arata V, Arduino PG, et al. Tooth extractions in intravenous bisphosphonate-treated patients: a refined protocol. J Oral Maxillofac Surg 2013;71:994–9.

78. Mavrokokki T, Cheng A, Stein B, et al. Nature and frequency of bisphosphonate-associated osteonecrosis of the jaws in Australia. J Oral Maxillofac Surg 2007;65:415–23.

79. Regev E, Lustmann J, Nashef R. Atraumatic teeth extraction in bisphosphonate-treated patients. J Oral Maxillofac Surg 2008;66:1157–61.

80. Smidt A, Lipovetsky-Adler M, Sharon E. Forced eruption as an alternative to tooth extraction in long-term use of oral bisphosphonates. J Am Dent Assoc 2012;143:1303–12.

81. Tsao C, Darby I, Ebeling PR, et al. Oral health risk factors for bisphosphonates-associated osteonecrosis. J Oral Maxillofac Surg 2013;71: 1360–6.

Oral Surgery in Patients Undergoing Chemoradiation Therapy

Nagi M. Demian, DDS, MD[a,b,*], Jonathan W. Shum, DDS, MD[c], Ivan L. Kessel, MD[d], Ahmed Eid, MD[e]

KEYWORDS

• Cancer • Chemotherapy • Head and neck radiation therapy • Interruption • Oral surgery
• Oral complications

KEY POINTS

- Despite advances in therapies for cancers, oral and dental care and prevention still lagging in patients with cancer.
- Oral and maxillofacial surgeons treating patients with cancer face diverse and numerous chemotherapy and radiation protocols.
- Delays or interruption in chemotherapy or radiation therapy delivery can adversely affect the prognosis and survival of patients with cancer.
- Familiarity with side effects, treatment cycle durations, blood count nadirs, and recovery periods are critical.
- Best outcomes are delivered via a multidisciplinary approach.

Comprehensive oral care in the patient with head and neck cancer remains a challenge, because many such patients have undergone surgical therapy and/or radiotherapy with or without chemotherapy. Each treatment modality brings posttherapy changes to the patients' physiology and anatomy that can significantly affect the management of otherwise routine dental procedures and oral hygiene. As a part of a multidisciplinary approach, the oral and maxillofacial surgeon (OMFS) attempts to address these changes while providing care to avoid problems that can adversely affect the patient's quality of life, such as osteoradionecrosis (ORN), trismus, and xerostomia.[1,2]

Many factors influence the way cancer is treated. Geographic location can influence the availability of multiple specialists; fear and economic factors can deter patients from seeking care early, leading to late presentation and urgency in delivering therapies to treat metastatic cancer. In those compromised situations in which there is limited time available before the start of treatment, patients with cancer may be adversely affected by the lack of adequate preparations and the lack of a multidisciplinary approach. In

[a] Oral & Maxillofacial Surgery Department, The University of Texas School of Dentistry, Lyndon B. Johnson Hospital, UT Annex 112 B, 5656 Kelly, Houston, TX 77026, USA; [b] The Externship Program, Dental Branch at UTHSC, UT Annex 112 B, 5656 Kelly, Houston, TX 77026, USA; [c] Department of Oral and Maxillofacial Surgery, University of Texas Health Science Center at Houston, 7500 Cambridge Street, Suite 6510, Houston, TX 77054, USA; [d] Department of Radiation Oncology, University of Texas Medical Branch, 301 University Boulevard, Galveston, TX 77555, USA; [e] General Oncology, The University of Texas MD Anderson Cancer Center, 1515 Holcombe Boulevard, Unit 0462, Houston, TX 77030, USA
* Corresponding author. Oral & Maxillofacial Surgery Department, The University of Texas Dental Branch, Lyndon B. Johnson Hospital, UT Annex 112 B, 5656 Kelly, Houston, TX 77026.
E-mail address: nagi.demian@uth.tmc.edu

Oral Maxillofacial Surg Clin N Am 26 (2014) 193–207
http://dx.doi.org/10.1016/j.coms.2014.01.006
1042-3699/14/$ – see front matter © 2014 Elsevier Inc. All rights reserved.

addition, neutropenic fever risk and odontogenic abscesses, whether de novo or exacerbations of old conditions, may ensue, causing hardships and possible costly delays in chemotherapy or radiation therapy.

As such, consultations for dental clearance before the start of therapy have a complex myriad of factors to consider before, during, and after the completion of cancer treatment. Multidisciplinary care usually involves a tumor board or committee in which cancer cases are holistically discussed and input from every specialist is expected and heard. Coordinators usually arrange for the patients to be seen and treated individually. A head and neck tumor board typically involves an oncologist, a radiation oncologist, a head and neck surgeon, a maxillofacial prosthodontist, an oral and maxillofacial surgeon, a speech therapist, a social worker/case manager, a pathologist, a diagnostic radiologist, and a coordinator.

EPIDEMIOLOGY

Although the incidence of new cancer cases has decreased there were more than 1.5 to 1.6 million cases of cancer diagnosed in 2010. Lung, prostate, and colorectal cancer are the top 3 cancers in men, and breast followed by colorectal cancers in women.[3,4] About 3% of cancer cases involve the head and neck, and roughly 20% of those patients die each year.[3,4]

Because of the continuing decrease in public funding for routine adult dental care, and the inability of segments of society to afford private dental care because of economic difficulty, patients are increasingly relying on emergency rooms for their dental emergencies.[5]

Few dental providers are able to care for patients with cancer because of the complexity of their treatment. Hospital dentists, especially OMFSs, are often asked to consult, treat, and follow patients with cancer.

In a systematic review, Hong and colleagues[6] found that the prevalence of decayed, missing, and filled teeth is highest among patients who have received radiation therapy as a treatment modality for their cancer, whereas the highest prevalence of caries was among those who were treated with chemotherapy as the sole modality of treatment.

The difficulties discussed earlier present a challenge to OMFSs and any dentist treating patients with cancer because they need to keep abreast of the general principles of cancer therapies and their side effects and to communicate with all parties involved in the care of these patients to prevent avoidable oral complications and to improve outcomes.

CHEMOTHERAPY

Conventional cytotoxic chemotherapy uses agents that work by targeting rapidly dividing cells by interfering with DNA synthesis or by damaging their cellular infrastructure. Some are cell cycle specific and others are not. However, these cytotoxic agents do not differentiate between tumor cells and normal cells. Chemotherapy is given with 2 main intents: cure and palliation. It can be given to treat persistent tumor cells after surgery or radiation in what is known as adjuvant therapy. Neoadjuvant chemotherapy is given to reduce the tumor burden before definitive therapy. Chemotherapy and radiation are often delivered concurrently, the details of which can be found elsewhere in this issue. Chemotherapy may also be administered concurrently with radiation therapy, in which it is used as a sensitizer of tumor cells to radiation therapy.

Most cytotoxic chemotherapeutic agents result in myelosuppression. This is one of the most significant side effects that may influence the initiation of any surgical intervention. Other common side effects are fatigue, nausea, vomiting, mucositis, alopecia, organ damage, and loss or alteration of taste.[7]

The nonhematologic toxicities of most chemotherapy agents are acute, generally start on the first day of chemotherapy, and can last for 3 to 5 days. Hematologic toxicities such as leukopenia, anemia, and thrombocytopenia start after 5 to 7 days with the lowest blood count occurring at 10 to 14 days. This reduction in blood count is generally followed by bone marrow recovery. The nadir is deeper and longer for chemotherapy given for hematologic malignancies such as leukemia and after stem cell transplantation. Because chemotherapy is given in cycles to maximize cancer cell death while allowing the bone marrow cells to recover, knowing approximately when the nadir is expected and when recovery happens is crucial to selecting an appropriate time to perform needed dental and oral surgery procedures as safely as possible rather than causing unnecessary delays in treatment that can adversely affect treatment outcomes and patients' survival.[8]

RADIATION THERAPY

Through the transfer of high kinetic energy, radiation therapy causes direct disruption to molecular structures. Cell death occurs as a result of structural damage to the mechanisms of DNA synthesis. Although chemotherapy is systemic, radiation therapy is targeted at the primary tumor location, and/or the associated draining lymphatic nodal basin.

The gray (Gy) is the unit used to quantify the dose of energy and 1 Gy is equal to 1 J of energy absorbed in 1 kg of tissue.

Fractionation is the process of delivering small doses of radiation over more treatments (ie, 2 treatments vs 1 per day) until the total dose is achieved. Fractionation allows for some recovery of normal cells while achieving the desired tumor cell kill.[9]

Therapeutic radiation dose differs depending on the tumor site. In the head and neck region up to 70 Gy are required for the primary tumor site.

Efforts must be made to avoid interruptions in radiation therapy to avoid deleterious consequences on outcome and survival. In their review of more than 150 cases of oropharyngeal carcinomas, Allal and colleagues[10] found that interruption of radiation therapy was a significant independent adverse prognostic factor. Furthermore, studies have shown that a delay in the initiation of radiation therapy following surgery can be detrimental if it lasts longer than 6 weeks. Ideal radiation therapy should be completed in less than 13 weeks from surgery. Local regional control following surgery and radiation therapy is 62% at greater than 11 weeks versus 38% at greater than 13 weeks.[11]

PREPARATIONS BEFORE THE START OF THERAPY

A thorough understanding of the patient's disease, treatment plan, and prognosis is crucial.

The Patient Receiving Chemotherapy

- As noted earlier, chemotherapy kills rapidly dividing cells but also inhibits bone marrow precursor cells, leading to myelosuppression. Nadirs can reach levels consistent with severe neutropenia (<500 neutrophils) and patients on chemotherapy can develop mucositis and are prone to bacterial infections.
- A thorough discussion must be had with the patient explaining the side effects and potential complications of chemotherapy.
- Careful evaluation of the patient's oral cavity, with radiographic imaging, periodontal screening, and assessment of existing restorations and for incidental maxillofacial disorders, must be completed routinely.
- Careful consideration for the patients' ability to care for their own dentition based on individual patient history and willingness to adhere to recommendations.
- Extract hopeless teeth, perform alveoplasty, obtain primary closure, and allow surgical sites to heal adequately before the start of therapy. Exactly how long to wait after oral surgery, especially extraction of teeth, and the start of therapy is not as important as a clinical finding of adequate healing based on history and a careful examination. It can range from 10 days[12] to 6 weeks.[13]
- Stop the use of ill-fitting dentures and prostheses, and consider implant placements for improvement of prosthetic stability in patients about to start systemic bisphosphonate or other antiresorptive therapies such as the receptor activator of nuclear factor kappa-B ligand (RANKL) monoclonal antibody denosumab. One of the causes of osteonecrosis secondary to these drugs is loose or ill-fitting prostheses or dentures,[2] which can result in trauma to the oral mucosa and can expose the underlying bone. Placement of dental implants therefore can benefit patients by reducing mobility of their prostheses and improving their quality of life.
- Caries control and elimination.
- Periodontal disease control with scaling and root planning.
- Fluoride therapy.
- Meticulous oral hygiene enforced by frequent follow-up visits every 3 months.
- Most importantly, establishing an excellent rapport with patients and gaining their trust, and assuring them that the provider is available to assist them with their difficulties and complications.

The Patient Receiving Radiation to the Head and Neck Region

The same recommendations apply (**Table 1**).

The main difference between the effects of radiation and the effects of chemotherapy is that the latter are mostly temporary.

In addition to the immediate and direct damage that radiation therapy inflicts on the structures in the head and neck region, there is a potentially more serious and delayed injury that affects that same region. Radiation can greatly reduce the irradiated patients' quality of life because of side effects such as mucositis, radiation-induced fibrosis, trismus, xerostomia, and dysgeusia.

Popular theories of ORN are driven by the sequence of events that follow persistent tissue hypoxia leading to hypocellularity and hypovascularity.[14] Contemporary understanding of ORN suggests the progression of ORN to be the activation and dysregulation of fibroblastic activity that leads to atrophic tissue within an irradiated area. To address this aspect of ORN new management regimens have been developed that include the use of

Table 1
Recommended preparation before start of therapy

Type of Therapy	Tumor Board	Dental/Prosthodontic Evaluation	Oral and Maxillofacial Surgeon
Chemotherapy	Diagnosis Treatment plan Prognosis	Oral examination and history DMFT Periodontal examination and probing Dental radiographs Dental hygiene Fluoride treatment: 1.1% sodium fluoride gel or 0.4% stannous fluoride if no mucositis present Follow-up every 3 mo	Remove all hopeless, diseased teeth Perform alveoplasty, remove all bony protuberances or sharp spots Consider placement of dental implants for prosthetic support Postoperative follow-up until healing (minimum of 3 wk before therapy)
RT to the head and neck	Diagnosis Treatment plan Prognosis Dose map of RT	Oral examination and history DMFT Periodontal examination and probing Dental radiographs Dental hygiene Fluoride treatment: 1.1% sodium fluoride gel or 0.4% stannous fluoride if no mucositis present Follow-up every 3 mo Oral positioning or shielding devices	Remove all hopeless, diseased teeth; teeth exposed to >60 Gy Perform alveoplasty, remove all bony protuberances or sharp spots Consider placement of dental implants for prosthetic support Establish MIO Start jaw-stretching exercise regimen Consider coronoidectomy Postoperative follow-up until healing (minimum of 3 wk before therapy)

Abbreviations: DMFT, decayed, missing or filled teeth; MIO, maximal interincisor opening; RT, radiation therapy.

pentoxifylline with tocopherol. These agents inhibit the proliferation of fibroblasts and also scavenge the reactive oxygen species that are secondary to radiation damage.[15]

The dose of radiation delivered mediates the incidence and severity of ORN, which is more prevalent in regions that have received more than 60 Gy. However, the incidence of ORN is thought to be less common after hyperfractionated radiotherapy up to 72 to 80 Gy.[16] The combination with chemotherapy is thought to increase the incidence of ORN, whereas the use of intensity-modulated radiotherapy (IMRT) may reduce it.[17]

Knowledge of the approximate radiation field to the head and neck is therefore essential to identify the areas that will receive greater than a 60-Gy dose of radiation (**Fig. 1**).

The debate over the cause of dental caries after radiation continues, with few clinicians still claiming that the sole cause is radiation xerostomia. In their retrospective study evaluating teeth after radiation exposure, Walker and colleagues[18] found that those teeth exposed to more than 60 Gy had 10 times the odds of moderate to severe damage compared with teeth that had had no radiation exposure.

Grotz and colleagues[19] noted direct damage at the dentin-enamel junction and subsurface decay

in teeth exposed to more than 60 Gy in an in vitro study.

Teeth in areas expected to receive high doses of radiation, teeth with questionable disorders such as periapical radiolucencies, and teeth with large restorations and questionable margins must be removed.

Consideration must be given to rehabilitation and elimination of possible causes of ORN, such as ill-fitting dentures, by placement of dental implants preferably in areas not planned to receive high doses of radiation. Schoen and colleagues[20] found that there was no significant difference in success of patients who were restored prosthetically with dentoalveolar implants placed before treatment and who had undergone radiotherapy versus patients who were not treated with radiotherapy.

Customized prostheses to protect normal tissue from radiation are vital in reducing morbidities and severe side effects from radiation. These oral appliances displace and shield normal tissue from the effects of radiation. Fabrication of these custom devices must be a part of the overall preparation before the start of radiation therapy for the head and neck region (**Fig. 2**).[21,22] These appliances are custom fabricated with acrylic similarly

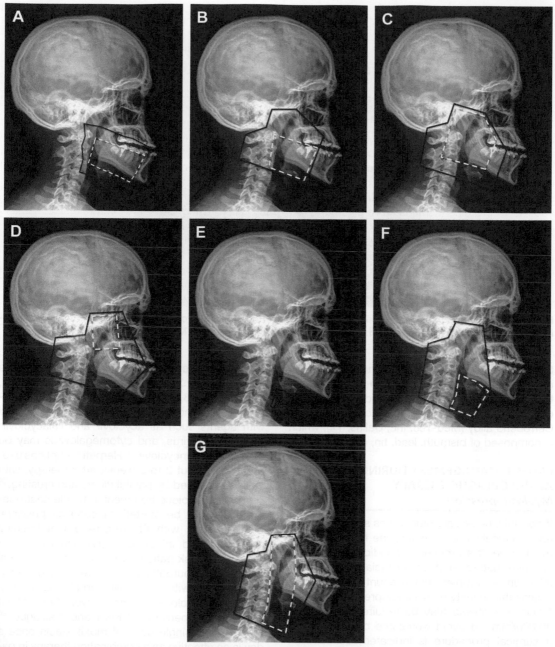

Fig. 1. Approximate radiation doses to the mandible and maxilla in common head and neck cancers. Conformation with IMRT for three-dimensional assessment and laterality is mandatory. Consultation with a radiation oncologist is vital because the doses and areas exposed may change depending on tumor type and size. Solid black lines depict areas receiving more than 55 Gy and yellow dashed lines depict areas receiving more than 60 Gy. (*A*) Oral tongue and floor of the mouth. (*B*) Base of the tongue. (*C*) Posterior palate and tonsilar fossa. (*D*) Nasopharynx. (*E*) Vocal cords. (*F*) Larynx. (*G*) Posterior pharyngeal wall. (*Modified from* Ang K, Garden AS. Radiotherapy for head and neck cancers. 4th edition. Philadelphia: Lippincott Williams & Wilkins; 2012; and Beumer J, Curtis TA, Marunick MT. Maxillofacial rehabilitation, prosthodontic and surgical consideration. Saint Louis (MO): Ishiyaku EuroAmerica; 1996.)

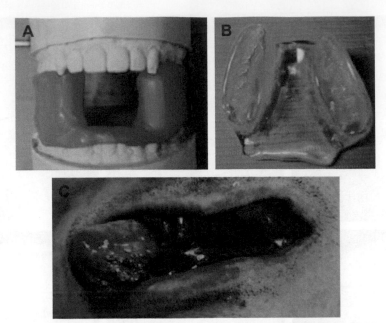

Fig. 2. Custom oral radiation prosthesis. (*A*) Custom fabrication. (*B*) Final prosthesis. (*C*) Prosthesis in place displacing tongue out of the radiation field. (*Courtesy of* Joann Marruffo, DDS, MS, Houston, TX.)

to other dental prostheses, and, if needed, barriers made of protective materials can be embedded to protect certain areas from the side effects of radiation. An example of such protective material is Cerrobend alloy (Med-Tec, Inc, Dallas, TX), which is composed of bismuth, lead, tin, and cadmium.

PATIENT MANAGEMENT DURING ANTINEOPLASTIC THERAPY
Myelosuppression

If possible, necessary procedures should be done approximately 1 week before the following treatment cycle. If a procedure is indicated and is of an acute nature, such as for facial trauma or an infection, a complete blood count is required to assess the severity of myelosuppression. A transfusion of platelets may be required if less than 40,000/mm^3 to avoid worrisome bleeding.[13,23] If a surgical procedure is indicated, consultation with the treating medical oncologist is necessary to identify the nadir in the treatment and the therapy cycle timing and duration.

Opportunistic infections may flourish in these immune compromised patients and can be of bacterial, fungal, or viral origin. Treatment of these infections should be targeted to the relevant organism, as guided by cultures and antibiotic sensitivities.

Mucositis secondary to yeast infections such as candida, of which there are pseudomembranous and erythematous types, are treated with nystatin suspension and topical agents such as

miconazole. Severe candida infections should be treated with systemic agents such as fluconazole, amphotericin B, or antifungal agents. Herpes simplex virus 1 and varicella zoster virus are treated with agents such as acyclovir and valacyclovir. Epstein-Barr virus, and cytomegalovirus may be treated with gancyclovir.[13] Herpetic eruptions usually occur about 2 to 3 weeks after therapy, with vesicles followed by painful ulcers and crusting.[24]

Empiric antibiotic treatment in febrile neutropenia (FN) must be started as soon as possible. Most patients with FN require urgent hospital admission and intravenous (IV) antibiotics. For the few low-risk patients who can treated by oral antibiotics as outpatients, some recommend a fluoroquinolone with amoxicillin and clavulanic acid, or a fluoroquinolone with clindamycin if the patient is allergic to penicillin.[25] Kern and colleagues[26] found that a single dose of moxifloxacin once a day is as effective as a combination therapy in patients with low-risk FN.

Hematopoietic growth factors such as granulocyte colony-stimulating factors or granulocyte-macrophage colony-stimulating factors should be considered for prophylaxis and treatment of FN.[27]

Mucositis

Mucositis of the oral cavity is a common and serious side effect of chemotherapy and radiation therapy. It results in severe pain, difficulty in feeding and hydrating, decreases the patient's ability to maintain good oral hygiene, and ultimately may delay or interrupt therapy, which may adversely affect survival and prognosis.[24,28] Mucositis is graded by the World Health Organization criteria from 1 to 4 depending on its severity; from mild soreness in grade 1 to a large painful ulcer with difficulty tolerating oral intake in grade 4.[24] The severity and duration of oral mucositis is related to the severity of neutropenia, the agents used, the dosing of the cytotoxic agent, or the dose of radiation.

The mucosal injury is thought to occur through a sequence of 5 events. The initial insult is the direct apoptotic effect of the antineoplastic therapy, which starts about 4 to 7 days after the beginning of therapy. A second indirect effect occurs with the upregulation of multiple inflammatory cytokines such as tumor necrosis factor alpha, interleukin-1β, and interleukin-6. The third stage is the amplification of the second stage leading to the generation of more inflammatory cytokines and leading to a fourth, ulcerative stage (**Fig. 3**). Evidence of healing and recovery mark the fifth phase.[13,24,28]

Microbial agents (fungal, viral, and bacterial) discussed earlier can worsen and lengthen the duration of mucositis, and therefore timely intervention and treatment are important.

Many combinations of rinses and different agents are recommended (**Table 2**). However, there is a lack of evidence to support specific oral rinse regimens regarding their efficacy in the reduction of mucositis or oral infections after chemotherapy or radiation therapy.[24,28]

Saline rinses with or without baking soda are preferred to more expensive and possibly irritating mixes, especially because many of the different mixes also known as magic mouth washes or miracle mouth washes containing agents like diphenhydramine and lidocaine have shown no advantage compared with basic saline and baking soda rinses.[29]

The common chlorhexidine (CHX) rinses come in a 0.12% solution that contains alcohol. Alcohol may be an irritant for patients with mucositis.

Another controversy about the use of CHX is the suggested increased susceptibility to gram-negative bacteria (GNB) infections especially after bone marrow transplant (BMT). After an extensive review of the available literature, Raybould and colleagues[30] found that GNB infections in patients receiving BMT occur regardless of the use of CHX. CHX rinse, preferably in an alcohol-free preparation, may be considered because of its broad-spectrum antibacterial coverage and its antifungal properties.

Other agents such as sucralfate, topical viscous lidocaine, diphenhydramine, milk of magnesium, and topical steroids are used in combination or as single agents depending on the provider's experience or the individual institutions' protocols.

Care must be taken when topical anesthetics are used because these agents may cause hypoalimentation because of the unpleasant effects of altered taste and sensation in the oral cavity.[24] Systemic and effective analgesics must be considered for adequate pain control when mucositis is severe.

Cryotherapy before the start of chemotherapy (fluorouracil) infusion has been shown to be beneficial in reducing oral mucositis. Ice chips or frozen lozenges can be used 5 minutes before the infusion with good effect.[13,28]

Neurotoxicity and Taste Alteration

Some chemotherapeutic agents may cause direct nerve toxicity and can manifest as a pulsating mandibular pain despite there being no dental source. However, this symptom is self-limiting and subsides after chemotherapy.

Neurotoxicity can affect gustatory cells and cause alteration or loss of the sense of taste.

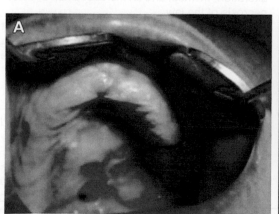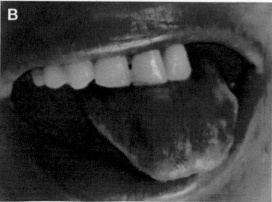

Fig. 3. (*A*) Severe mucositis 1 to 3 weeks after the start of radiation therapy. (*B*) Mucositis of the tongue may also affect taste. (*Courtesy of* Joann Marruffo, DDS, MS, Houston, TX.)

Table 2
Risk factors for ORN of the jaw bones and antiresorptive therapy–related necrosis of the jaw bones (AONJ)

	Therapy	Risk Factors	Incidence (%)
ORN	>60 Gy RT for head and neck cancer	Posterior mandible Proximity to tumor Poor oral hygiene Odontogenic disorder Ill-fitting prosthesis Trauma, including surgical	5–15 Decrease to 6 with IMRT and three-dimensional planning
AONJ	N-NB or monoclonal antibodies to RANKL	Duration of therapy Concomitant steroids or chemotherapy Mandible Poor oral hygiene Odontogenic disorder Ill-fitting prosthesis Trauma, including surgical	1.3–1.8 in patients undergoing antiresorptive therapy for metastatic cancer

Abbreviation: N-NB, nitrogen-containing bisphosphonates.
Data from Jacobson AS, Buchbinder D, Hu K, et al. Paradigm shifts in the management of osteoradionecrosis of the mandible. Oral Oncol 2010;46(11):795–801; and Yamashita J, McCauley LK. Antiresorptives and osteonecrosis of the jaw. J Evid Based Dent Pract 2012;12(Suppl 3):233–47.

Dysgeusia also subsides after the conclusion of chemotherapy. Xerostomia and radiation effect can prolong the taste alteration or loss. Patients can have permanent alteration or loss of taste after chemoradiation therapy.[13]

Xerostomia

Patients can begin experiencing dry mouth 1 or 2 weeks after irradiation of the major salivary glands (parotid, submandibular, and sublingual). In 7 weeks the salivary flow decreases by about 80%. Damage to the fibrovascular stroma, loss of stem cells, and the lack of a regenerative response reflect the effect of radiation to the salivary system.[31] Recovery of salivary function is unlikely at doses of radiation higher than 64 Gy.[28]

Along with alterations to taste and speech, patients with xerostomia have difficulty chewing and swallowing solid and dry food, and their oral mucosa becomes fragile and susceptible to infections and trauma leading to mucositis.[31]

Drinking ample water, choosing bland, non-spicy, and soft food, and avoiding removable prosthesis wear are some of the adjustments the patient may have to make.

A dose of radiation less than 26 Gy is suggested to the parotid gland to preserve most of its function.[31]

Amifostine is a radiation-protective agent for the salivary gland and may reduce the degree of post-radiation xerostomia. It functions as a scavenger to H+ ions, neutralizes oxygen radicals, and prevents oxidative damage if administered immediately before each fraction of radiation therapy.[28,31]

Pilocarpine is a cholinergic agonist that stimulates salivary production at dosages of 5 mg orally 3 to 4 times per day. A topical form can also be used with equal effectiveness and fewer side effects.[28]

Artificial saliva, sugarless candies, and sugar-free xylitol-containing chewing gum are all recommended adjuncts in addition to high-water-content foods to help minimize the adverse effects of xerostomia on the quality of life of patients.[13,28,31]

AFTER CHEMOTHERAPY AND RADIATION THERAPY

Patients who have received head and neck radiation may have long-term xerostomia and taste alteration, trismus, and an increased risk of osteonecrosis of the jaw.

Patients who receive antiresorptive treatment such as bisphosphonates or antibody to RANKL may also be at risk for developing necrosis of the jaws.

Trismus

One of the most frustrating complications of head and neck cancer is trismus, which most frequently is caused by tumors but may also result from surgery or radiation therapy to the head and neck region. The fibrosis of the masticator muscles can occur secondary to radiation and/or surgical intervention for tumors involving the masseter or the pterygoid muscles (**Fig. 4**). Any new-onset trismus in the patient with head and neck cancer during

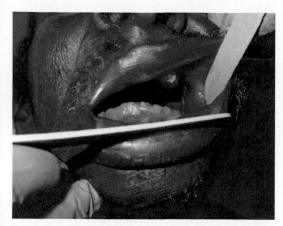

Fig. 4. Severe trismus after surgical ablation of a tumor involving the posterior maxilla and retromolar trigone, followed by radiation therapy. No concomitant coronoidectomy was performed.

surveillance should alert clinicians to the possibility of recurrent disease.[32]

Physical therapy to improve mouth opening should be reviewed with patients before treatment, especially if treatment involves the area of the masticator muscles or the coronoid area. Jaw-stretching exercises can limit the amount of trismus in the postoperative period. Manual manipulation is a simple and inexpensive technique that involves the use of patients' own fingers to forcibly open their mouths or to stack tongue depressors; these are classic ways to train jaw function. Maximal interincisor opening (MIO) should be recorded to monitor progress and compliance with treatment.

When trismus is confirmed to be of a nonneoplastic origin, stretching exercises can be started at least 4 times daily with a 1-mm daily MIO improvement goal.[28] Commercially available mechanical

devices can be helpful. Stubblefield and colleagues[33] found that patients with head and neck cancer with trismus showed more substantial improvement in their MIOs when they complied with dynamic jaw-opening exercises using devices such as Dynasplint than patients using other methods.

However, despite physical therapy and other forms of management, trismus in patients with head and neck cancer remains difficult to treat.[34]

Coronoidectomy (**Fig. 5**) can significantly improve trismus by releasing the fibrotic attachment of the temporalis muscle and removing the coronoid process.[35] However, following surgical ablation, reconstruction, and radiation therapy, additional surgery may be required to cover defects resulting from the coronoidectomy procedure. Mardini and colleagues[36] described their approach of free vascularized flap reconstruction after release of trismus in patients previously treated for head and neck cancer and reconstructed with additional vascularized free flap reconstruction.

There is an increased risk of ORN after a procedure such as coronoidectomy in areas exposed to high doses of radiation. Clinicians should give considerations to performing coronoidectomy procedures when the ascending ramus is within the radiation field or adjacent to the site of surgical ablation. In patients who receive nonsurgical definitive treatment, caution must be exercised to ensure that coronoidectomy does not violate oncologic principles (ie, incision through the tumor).

PREVENTION AND TREATMENT OF OSTEONECROSIS OF THE JAW BONE

In patients with cancer, osteonecrosis of the jaw (ONJ) generally manifests as an exposed area of

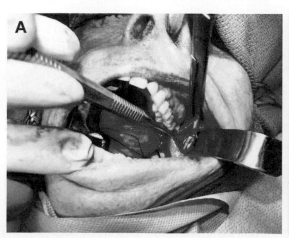
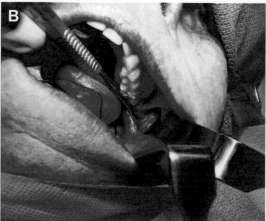

Fig. 5. (*A*) Exposure of the coronoid and release of the temporalis muscle attachment. (*B*) After removal of the coronoid process.

bone that has received more than a 60-Gy dose of radiation or in a patient who has undergone antiresorptive therapy with nitrogen-containing bisphosphonates (N-BP) or monoclonal antibodies to RANKL such as denosumab. The first of these is commonly referred to as ORN and the last is referred to as antiresorptive osteonecrosis of the jaws (AONJ). The term bisphosphonate-related AONJ was previously used rather than AONJ; however, recent studies suggest that agents other than bisphosphonates can also instigate osteonecrosis. ORN is diagnosed when the exposure is for more than 3 months and when cancer recurrence has been ruled out. AONJ is diagnosed when the bone is exposed for 8 weeks with no history of radiation or cancer (**Fig. 6**).

Pathophysiology of ORN is described earlier as proliferation of radiation-induced fibrosis and obliteration of blood vessels leading to hypoxia, hypocellularity, and hypovascularity of the jaws, as opposed to AONJ, which is the result of reduced bone turnover caused by osteoclast inactivity or differentiation.[14,37–41]

The incidence of ORN is 5% to 15 % in areas of the jaws exposed to more than 60 Gy.[38] The incidence of AONJ in patients undergoing antiresorptive therapy with metastatic disease is 1.8% for those treated with denosumab and 1.3% for those treated with N-BP.[42]

Many of the risk factors for both entities are similar, such as odontogenic and periodontal disorders, dentoalveolar surgery, trauma to oral tissue (such as in the presence of large tori or other bony protuberances), and ill-fitting prosthesis (see **Table 2**).[2,38]

There is an in-depth discussion of the surgical treatment of antiresorptive therapy–induced osteonecrosis of the jaw elsewhere in this issue.

Oral Surgery in Irradiated Jaws

A problem facing dentists and oral surgeons is how to address an indicated oral surgical procedure such an extraction of a painful nonrestorable tooth, treatment of an abscess, or even a mandible fracture in the patient with irradiated head and neck cancer. The concern is the instigation of ORN. ORN in areas exposed to less than 60 Gy is unlikely. In addition, the use of IMRT and fractionation has further decreased the incidence of ORN.[41] Knowledge of the radiation field allows better oral care so indicated procedures can be performed for areas that are exposed to doses less than 50 Gy. However, despite all these advances, if the patient presents without the appropriate information and documentation of the received treatment and radiation dose map, 2 things can happen: delay in needed treatment and unnecessary and costly prophylactic therapies, or procedures performed in areas of high radiation exposure causing ORN. Another issue is the cost of the appropriate treatment. This issue applies to a patient told that an extraction of a painful tooth is not safe and that root canal therapy and a restoration or a coronectomy are needed for a nonrestorable tooth, which they cannot afford, leading to the patient searching for a provider who will remove the abnormal tooth to help relieve the patient's pain.

Avoidance of a procedure such as extraction of a tooth in an area irradiated with more than 60 Gy does not eliminate the risk of ORN because the pulpal disorder and possibly the abscess can still cause it.

Prophylactic Hyperbaric Oxygen Therapy

In a study involving the trial of prophylactic hyperbaric oxygen (HBO) therapy in patients who had

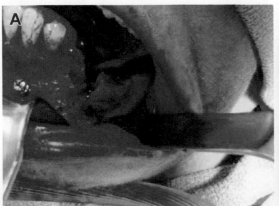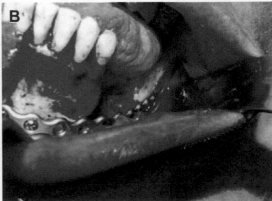

Fig. 6. (*A*) Pathologic fracture caused by AONJ in a patient with bone metastasis from a breast cancer. She was treated with IV N-BP. Presentation is 1 year after a nonhealing dental extraction site. (*B*) After debridement and reconstruction with a titanium reconstruction plate.

received high doses of radiation to the head and neck region, Marx and colleagues[43] reported a significant decrease in the incidence of ORN in the pre-extraction HBO prophylactic treatment group compared with pre-extraction penicillin: 5.4% versus 29.9% respectively (**Fig. 7**). The protocol involves 20 pre-extraction dives at 2.4 times the atmospheric pressure in 100% oxygen for 90 minutes per dive followed by 10 dives after extraction. The technique has some side effects, such as ear barotrauma. The benefit comes from the angiogenesis that is induced after the creation of a gradient of oxygen tension between normal and hypoxic irradiated tissue. Macrophages usually follow the new blood supply and enhance healing.

Many clinicians have questioned the validity of that study and the efficacy of the approach.[44]

Despite the scrutiny, HBO is still offered if there is no contraindication to its use and if it is available.[12]

There is no evidence that HBO has any effect on tumor growth or metastasis.[45,46]

Other medical and pharmacologic modalities to treat ORN, such pentoxifylline and tocopherol, are discussed elsewhere in this issue.

ORN: Classification and Treatment

Stage 1 ORN involves a superficial exposure of bone for 3 months. Treatment involves local wound treatment and light debridement followed by 20 to 30 HBO dives. If there is response and improvement the patient receives an additional 10 HBO dives. If there is no improvement then the classification becomes stage 2.

Stage 2 ORN involves deeper layers, and wound debridement of all necrotic tissues until viable hard and soft tissues are reached. Tension-free closure with healthy mucosa must be accomplished. If soft tissue closure is not possible then vascularized soft tissue sift as rotational flaps or free vascularized flaps are needed to achieve complete closure (**Fig. 8**).

Stage 3 ORN is usually a full-thickness disease and presents with a pathologic fracture, fistula, or both. Complete resection of necrotic bone and soft tissue must be performed. Vascularized soft tissue and hard tissue transfer is usually needed to adequately reconstruct the residual defect (**Fig. 9**).

Dental Implant Placement After Radiation Therapy to the Head and Neck Region

Caution is needed when considering surgical procedures after radiation therapy, especially in edentulous patients with cancer. After ablation and reconstruction, the inability to function can have a severe adverse effect on the patient's quality of life and the ability to eat and interact socially. Prosthetic rehabilitation should be kept reasonable and allow for examination of underlying tissue. Therefore implant-supported overdentures are the best prostheses that allow cancer surveillance, are cost effective, are easy to clean, and do not require extensive surgical preparation or a large number of implants. Two successfully osseointegrated implants allow reasonable stability of the prosthesis. Placement of dental implants in the mandible is preferred in the interforamina anterior region where the radiation dose is usually lower

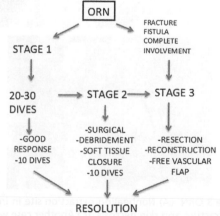

Fig. 7. Preventative and therapeutic use of HBO therapy.

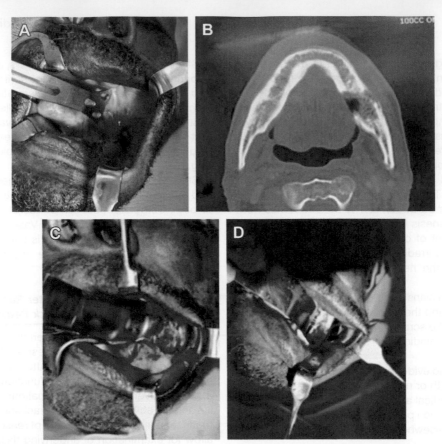

Fig. 8. Stage 2 ORN. (*A*) Nonhealing exposed bone after dental extraction in a previously irradiated mandible. Recurrence work-up was negative. HBO delivered with no response. (*B*) Bone necrosis deeper than first expected. (*C*) Necrotic bone exposed. (*D*) Removal of necrotic bone until vital bone was reached.

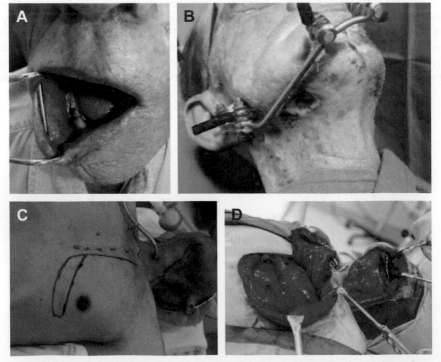

Fig. 9. Stage 3 ORN. (*A*) Nonhealing extraction site in irradiated mandible. (*B*) The condition has progressed to pathologic fracture and skin necrosis. (*C*) Another case with stage 3 ORN with pathologic fracture also following dental extraction. (*D*) Resulting defect requiring a transfer of vascularized tissue in the form of a pectoralis flap, skin paddle, and pedicled rib graft.

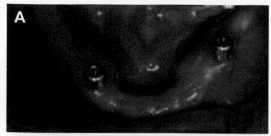

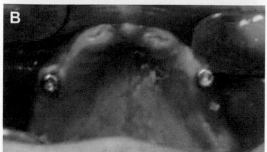

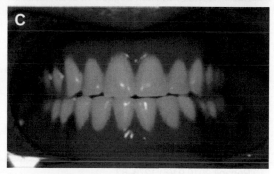

Fig. 10. (*A, B*) Two osseointegrated dental implants, in the mandible and maxilla respectively; note the healthy oral mucosa. (*C*) Stable implant-supported overdenture prosthesis. (*Courtesy of* Joann Marruffo, DDS, MS, Houston, TX.)

than in the posterior areas of the mandible (**Fig. 10**).[47]

In a systematic review, Colella and colleagues[48] found that there was no difference in the rate of implant failure between those placed before radiation therapy and those placed after radiation therapy, and found no implant failure if implants were placed in areas exposed to less than 45 Gy.

SUMMARY

Oral health care in patients undergoing chemotherapy and/or radiation therapy can be complex. Care delivered by a multidisciplinary approach is timely and streamlines the allocation of resources to provide prompt care and to attain favorable outcomes. A hospital dentist, oral and maxillofacial surgeon, and a maxillofacial prosthodontist must be involved early to prevent avoidable oral complications. Prevention and thorough preparation are vital before the start of chemotherapy and radiation therapy. Oral complications must be addressed immediately and, even with the best management, can cause delays and interruption in treatment, with serious consequences for the outcome and prognosis.

REFERENCES

1. Epstein JB, Thariat J, Bensadoun RJ, et al. Oral complications of cancer and cancer therapy: from cancer treatment to survivorship. CA Cancer J Clin 2012;62(6):400–22.
2. Yamashita J, McCauley LK. Antiresorptives and osteonecrosis of the jaw. J Evid Based Dent Pract 2012;12(Suppl 3):233–47.
3. Siegel R, Naishadham D, Jemal A. Cancer statistics, 2013. CA Cancer J Clin 2013;63(1):11–30.
4. Jemal A, Siegel R, Xu J, et al. Cancer statistics, 2010. CA Cancer J Clin 2010;60(5):277–300.
5. Wall T. Recent trends in dental emergency department visits in the United States: 1997/1998 to 2007/2008. J Public Health Dent 2012;72(3):216–20.
6. Hong CH, Napenas JJ, Hodgson BD, et al. A systematic review of dental disease in patients undergoing cancer therapy. Support Care Cancer 2010;18(8):1007–21.
7. Rosenthal PE. Complications of cancer treatment. Atlanta (GA): American Cancer Society; 2001.
8. Motzer RJ, Geller NL, Bosl GJ. The effect of a 7-day delay in chemotherapy cycles on complete response and event-free survival in good-risk disseminated germ cell tumor patients. Cancer 1990;66(5):857–61.
9. Mieszkalski G, Brady LW, Yeager TE, et al. Basis for current major therapies for cancer. Atlanta, GA: American Cancer Society; 2001.
10. Allal AS, de Pree C, Dulguerov P, et al. Avoidance of treatment interruption: an unrecognized benefit of accelerated radiotherapy in oropharyngeal carcinomas? Int J Radiat Oncol Biol Phys 1999;45(1): 41–5.
11. Ang KK, Trotti A, Brown BW, et al. Randomized trial addressing risk features and time factors of surgery plus radiotherapy in advanced head-and-neck cancer. Int J Radiat Oncol Biol Phys 2001; 51(3):571–8.
12. Kumar N, Brooke A, Burke M, et al. The oral management of oncology patients requiring radiotherapy, chemotherapy and / or bone marrow transplantation. Clinical guidelines. Updated 2012. London: The Royal College of Surgeons of England/The British Society for Disability and Oral Health; 2012.
13. López BC, Esteve CG, Pérez MG. Dental treatment considerations in the chemotherapy patient. J Clin Exp Dent 2011;3(1):e31–42.

14. Marx RE, Johnson RP. Studies in the radiobiology of osteoradionecrosis and their clinical significance. Oral Surg Oral Med Oral Pathol 1987;64(4):379–90.

15. Lyons A, Ghazali N. Osteoradionecrosis of the jaws: current understanding of its pathophysiology and treatment. Br J Oral Maxillofac Surg 2008;46(8):653–60.

16. Schwartz HC, Kagan AR. Osteoradionecrosis of the mandible: scientific basis for clinical staging. Am J Clin Oncol 2002;25(2):168–71.

17. Studer G, Studer SP, Zwahlen RA, et al. Osteoradionecrosis of the mandible: minimized risk profile following intensity-modulated radiation therapy (IMRT). Strahlenther Onkol 2006;182(5):283–8.

18. Walker MP, Wichman B, Cheng AL, et al. Impact of radiotherapy dose on dentition breakdown in head and neck cancer patients. Pract Radiat Oncol 2011;1(3):142–8.

19. Grotz KA, Duschner H, Kutzner J, et al. New evidence for the etiology of so-called radiation caries. Proof for directed radiogenic damage od the enamel-dentin junction. Strahlenther Onkol 1997;173(12):668–76.

20. Schoen P, Raghoebar G, Bouma J, et al. Prosthodontic rehabilitation of oral function in head-neck cancer patients with dental implants placed simultaneously during ablative tumour surgery: an assessment of treatment outcomes and quality of life. Int J Oral Maxillofac Surg 2008;37(1):8–16.

21. Poole T, Flaxman N. Use of protective prostheses during radiation therapy. J Am Dent Assoc 1986;112(4):485–8.

22. Fleming TJ, Rambach SC. A tongue-shielding radiation stent. J Prosthet Dent 1983;49(3):389–92.

23. Epstein J, Huber M, et al. Oral health in cancer therapy. A guide for health care professionals. In: Rankin KV, Jones DL, Redding SW, editors. 2008 Oral health in cancer therapy conference. San Antonio (TX): Cancer Prevention and Research Institute of Texas and Baylor Oral Health Foundation; 2008.

24. Köstler WJ, Hejna M, Wenzel C, et al. Oral mucositis complicating chemotherapy and/or radiotherapy: options for prevention and treatment. CA Cancer J Clin 2001;51(5):290–315.

25. Flowers CR, Seidenfeld J, Bow EJ, et al. Antimicrobial prophylaxis and outpatient management of fever and neutropenia in adults treated for malignancy: American Society of Clinical Oncology clinical practice guideline. J Clin Oncol 2013;31(6):794–810.

26. Kern WV, Marchetti O, Drgona L, et al. Oral antibiotics for fever in low-risk neutropenic patients with cancer: a double-blind, randomized, multicenter trial comparing single daily moxifloxacin with twice daily ciprofloxacin plus amoxicillin/clavulanic acid combination therapy–EORTC infectious diseases group trial XV. J Clin Oncol 2013;31(9):1149–56.

27. Gomez Raposo C, Pinto Marin A, Gonzalez Baron M. Colony-stimulating factors: clinical evidence for treatment and prophylaxis of chemotherapy-induced febrile neutropenia. Clin Transl Oncol 2006;8(10):729–34.

28. Sideras K, Loprinzi CL, Foote R. Oral complications of chemotherapy and radiation therapy. In: Laney W, Salinas T, Carr A, et al, editors. Diagnosis and treatment in prosthodontics. 2nd edition. Hanover (IL): Quintessence; 2011. p. 163–82.

29. Dodd MJ, Dibble SL, Miaskowski C, et al. Randomized clinical trial of the effectiveness of 3 commonly used mouthwashes to treat chemotherapy-induced mucositis. Oral Surg Oral Med Oral Pathol Oral Radiol Endod 2000;90(1):39–47.

30. Raybould TP, Carpenter AD, Ferretti GA, et al. Emergence of gram-negative bacilli in the mouths of bone marrow transplant recipients using chlorhexidine mouthrinse. Oncol Nurs Forum 1994;21(4):691–6.

31. Dirix P, Nuyts S, Van den Bogaert W, et al. Radiation-induced xerostomia in patients with head and neck cancer. Cancer 2006;107(11):2525–34.

32. Malis DD, Demian NM, Lemos L, et al. Carcinoid tumor presenting as trismus: immunohistochemical evidence of metastatic lung disease to the infratemporal fossa. J Oral Maxillofac Surg 2007;65(7):1382–8.

33. Stubblefield MD, Manfield L, Riedel ER. A preliminary report on the efficacy of a dynamic jaw opening device (Dynasplint Trismus System) as part of the multimodal treatment of trismus in patients with head and neck cancer. Arch Phys Med Rehabil 2010;91(8):1278–82.

34. Dijkstra P, Sterken M, Pater R, et al. Exercise therapy for trismus in head and neck cancer. Oral Oncol 2007;43(4):389–94.

35. Bhrany AD, Izzard M, Wood AJ, et al. Coronoidectomy for the treatment of trismus in head and neck cancer patients. Laryngoscope 2007;117(11):1952–6.

36. Mardini S, Chang Y-M, Tsai C-Y, et al. Release and free flap reconstruction for trismus that develops after previous intraoral reconstruction. Plast Reconstr Surg 2006;118(1):102–7.

37. Damm DD, Jones DM. Bisphosphonate-related osteonecrosis of the jaws: a potential alternative to drug holidays. Gen Dent 2013;61(5):33–8.

38. Jacobson AS, Buchbinder D, Hu K, et al. Paradigm shifts in the management of osteoradionecrosis of the mandible. Oral Oncol 2010;46(11):795–801.

39. McLeod NM, Bater MC, Brennan PA. Management of patients at risk of osteoradionecrosis: results of survey of dentists and oral & maxillofacial surgery units in the United Kingdom, and suggestions for best practice. Br J Oral Maxillofac Surg 2010;48(4):301–4.

40. Migliorati CA, Hsu CJ, Chopra S, et al. Dental management of patients with a history of bisphosphonate

therapy: clinical dilemma. J Calif Dent Assoc 2008; 36(10):769–74.

41. Nabil S, Samman N. Risk factors for osteoradionecrosis after head and neck radiation: a systematic review. Oral Surg Oral Med Oral Pathol Oral Radiol Endod 2012;113(1):54–69.

42. Saad F, Brown J, Van Poznak C, et al. Incidence, risk factors, and outcomes of osteonecrosis of the jaw: integrated analysis from three blinded active-controlled phase III trials in cancer patients with bone metastases. Ann Oncol 2012;23(5):1341–7.

43. Marx RE, Johnson RP, Kline SN. Prevention of osteoradionecrosis: a randomized prospective clinical trial of hyperbaric oxygen versus penicillin. J Am Dent Assoc 1985;111(1):49–54.

44. Fritz GW, Gunsolley JC, Abubaker O, et al. Efficacy of pre- and postirradiation hyperbaric oxygen therapy in the prevention of postextraction osteoradionecrosis: a systematic review. J Oral Maxillofac Surg 2010;68(11):2653–60.

45. Shi Y, Lee CS, Wu J, et al. Effects of hyperbaric oxygen exposure on experimental head and neck tumor growth, oxygenation, and vasculature. Head Neck 2005;27(5):362–9.

46. Narozny W, Kuczkowski J, Mikaszewski B. Radionecrosis or tumor recurrence after radiation: importance of choice for HBO. Otolaryngol Head Neck Surg 2007;137(1):176–7.

47. Dholam KP, Gurav SV. Dental implants in irradiated jaws: a literature review. J Cancer Res Ther 2012; 8(6):85.

48. Colella G, Cannavale R, Pentenero M, et al. Oral implants in radiated patients: a systematic review. Int J Oral Maxillofac Implants 2007;22(4):616.

Evaluation and Staging of the Neck in Patients with Malignant Disease

Jonathan W. Shum, DDS, MD[a],*, Eric J. Dierks, DMD, MD[b,c,d]

KEYWORDS

- Head and neck cancer • Neck evaluation • Neck staging • Neck imaging • PET • MRI • Ultrasound
- Squamous cell carcinoma

KEY POINTS

- Contemporary staging of cervical metastases relies on size and laterality of nodal involvement, with increasing size and number of nodal metastases representing higher stages of disease.
- The presence of a single metastatic lymph node reduces survival by 50%; the presence of bilateral cervical metastasis reduces survival by another 50%.
- Despite the identification of disease prior to overt clinical signs of recurrence, the mortality for salvage therapy remains high.

INTRODUCTION

Head and neck oncology encompasses a broad variety of entities that account for approximately 3% of all cancers in the United States.[1] There are more than 30 specific sites within the head and neck, of which cancer at each particular site is generally uncommon. Among all locations, the oral cavity and oropharynx are the sites that compose the large majority of cancers within the head and neck, of which 90% are squamous cell carcinoma (SCC).[2] Other malignant pathology includes salivary gland cancer, 2% to 4%, whereas melanoma, lymphoma, and sarcomas approximate 5%.[1] In most situations, the cancer does not originate from the structures of the neck; however, inherent to the nature of cancer, there is a tendency for regional and distant metastasis.

There are several routes for spread, including direct extension, lymphovascular drainage patterns, and via hematogenous routes. The prognostic impact of cervical metastasis is drastic; for example, in the context of SCC, survival is decreased by 50% with the discovery of a single metastatic ipsilateral lymph node and by another 50% if located in the contralateral neck.[3,4] Lindberg and, later, Shah described the predictable pattern of cervical metastasis of SCC in the head and neck, and diagnostic and treatment modalities have been refined to address the high-risk areas of spread.[5,6]

Current evaluation and staging of the neck include physical examination and imaging, such as CT, MRI, ultrasound (US), and positron emission tomography (PET). Contemporary staging of

Disclosures: We wish to confirm that there are no known conflicts of interest associated with this publication and there has been no significant financial support for this work that could have influenced its outcome.
[a] Department of Oral and Maxillofacial Surgery, University of Texas Health Science Center at Houston, 7500 Cambridge Street, Suite 6510, Houston, TX 77054, USA; [b] Trauma Service and Oral and Maxillofacial Surgery Service, Legacy Emanuel Medical Center, Portland, OR, USA; [c] Department of Oral and Maxillofacial Surgery, Oregon Health and Science University, Portland, OR, USA; [d] Head and Neck Surgical Associates, 1849 Northwest Kearney, Suite 300, Portland, OR 97209, USA
* Corresponding author.
E-mail address: jonathan.shum@uth.tmc.edu

Oral Maxillofacial Surg Clin N Am 26 (2014) 209–221
http://dx.doi.org/10.1016/j.coms.2014.01.007
1042-3699/14/$ – see front matter © 2014 Elsevier Inc. All rights reserved.

cervical metastases relies on size and laterality of nodal involvement, with increasing size and number of nodal metastases representing higher stages of disease. Advances in the understanding of cancer behavior have led to the recognition of extracapsular extension (ECE) in nodal disease as a significant poor prognostic feature independent from size.[7] Discussion is ongoing in regards to updating the current staging classification to incorporate the presence of ECE as part of tumor staging. Additional molecular markers (eg, human papillomavirus) and the extent of cellular differentiation have also been proposed to be incorporated into future updates for tumor classification and staging.

TNM CLASSIFICATION AND STAGING

After the diagnosis of a head and neck cancer, the stage of the tumor is determined through a complete physical examination in addition to the use of imaging techniques. The tumor-nodes-metastasis (TNM) classification is most widely used, endorsed and maintained by the American Joint Committee on Cancer (AJCC) and the Union for International Cancer Control (UICC). Since its introduction in 1968, the TNM staging system has stratified the severity of a cancer through the description of the anatomic extent of the primary tumor, regional lymph node involvement and presence of distant metastasis.[8] Variations of the TNM staging system exist in attempts to accommodate the variety of anatomic sites within the head and neck. **Table 1** outlines the criteria for nodal classification.[9] Lymphatic drainage patterns of the neck are classified into levels and defined by anatomic boundaries. **Fig. 1** illustrates the boundaries of the levels within the neck; **Table 2** describes the anatomic landmarks that define the boundaries of the neck. Generally, the progression of cervical disease spreads in a predictable direction through the levels of the neck and depends on the location of the primary tumor. Shah described these likely areas of cervical metastasis in SCC of the oral cavity as occurring more commonly in levels I to III; however, skip metastasis are a possibility but less likely.[10] The presence of advanced nodal disease (N >2a) increases the incidence of distant metastasis to as high as 46.8% when 3 or more cervical lymph nodes are involved.[3] Accurate evaluation of the neck is critical in establishing the correct stage to tailor primary and possible adjunctive therapy.

Information gathered from the physical examination and imaging studies is used to assign an initial clinical stage (cTNM). This classification directs patients toward the appropriate therapy

Table 1
TNM classification: criteria for neck staging
NX   Data unavailable
N0   No clinical or radiographic signs of regional node metastasis
N1   Cervical metastasis identified in ONE ipsilateral lymph node AND <3 cm in greatest dimension
N2a   Cervical metastasis identified in a single ipsilateral lymph node AND is >3 cm but <6 cm in greatest dimension
N2b   Cervical metastasis identified in multiple ipsilateral lymph nodes AND is <6 cm in greatest dimension
N2c   Cervical metastasis identified in bilateral or contralateral lymph nodes AND is <6 cm in greatest dimension
N3   Cervical metastasis identified in a lymph node >6 cm in greatest dimension

Modified from Edge S, Byrd DR, Compton CC, et al, editors. AJCC cancer staging manual. 7th edition. Springer Science and Business Media; 2010.

and provides prognostic information. Patients who undergo surgery are reassessed by means of a pathologic staging (pTNM) as determined by histopathology features from the final specimens obtained. This usually accounts for the primary tumor and, if applicable, the associated neck dissection(s). The results of the final pathology can modify the staging and ultimately the management and prognosis of the patient. Stage migration is a term that describes the potential false positive or

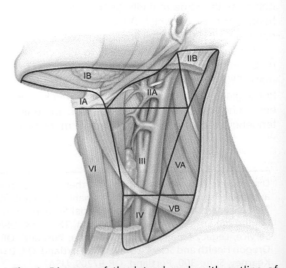

Fig. 1. Diagram of the lateral neck with outline of levels I–VI. (*From* Baredes S, Cohen E. The role of neck dissection in cancer of the oral cavity. Operat Tech Otolaryngol Head Neck Surg 2004;15:264.)

Table 2
Levels of the neck: anatomic boundaries

| Level | Group | Boundary | | | |
		Anterior	Posterior	Superior	Inferior
IA	Submental	Anterior belly of digastric m. (bilateral)	Mylohyoid	Mandible	Hyoid
IB	Submandibular	Anterior belly of digastric m.	Stylohyoid m.	Mandible	Posterior belly of digastric m.
IIA IIB	Upper jugular	Stylohyoid m. Spinal accessory n.	Spinal accessory n. Posterior border of SCM	Skull base	Hyoid
III	Middle jugular	Sternohyoid m.	Sensory branches of cervical plexus, medial to SCM	Hyoid	Cricoid
IV	Lower Jugular	Sternohyoid m.	Sensory branches of cervical plexus, medial to SCM	Cricoid	Clavicle
VA	Posterior triangle	Posterior border of SCM or sensory branches of cervical plexus	Trapezius m.	Convergence between SCM and trapezius	Cricoid
VB				Cricoid	Clavicle
VI	Anterior compartment	Contents anterior to common carotid artery		Hyoid	Suprasternal notch

Abbreviation: m, muscle; n, nerve; SCM, sternocleidomastoid.
Data from Robbins KT, Clayman G, Levine PA, et al. Neck dissection classification update: revisions proposed by the American Head and Neck Society and the American Academy of Otolaryngology-Head and Neck Surgery. Arch Otolaryngol Head Neck Surg 2002;128(7):751–8.

false negative findings that may occur between clinical and pathologic staging. The use of physical examination and imaging studies to interrogate the neck are subject to discrepancies that may be discovered following the examination of the pathologic specimen. A patient who was initially a cT2N0M0, stage 2, oral tongue SCC, undergoes surgery to reveal a pathology specimen with a tumor size of 4.5 cm and evidence of occult neck disease in 2 subcentimeter nodes. These findings upstage the patient to pT3N2bM0, stage 4, altering prognosis and management from surgery alone to surgery with adjuvant chemotherapy and radiation. Upstaging by pathology is not uncommon because occult cervical metastasis in a clinically negative neck ranges from 24% to 49%.[11–13] Stage may also change depending on the aggressiveness of the cancer. More often than not, patients can experience a lag period between consultation and treatment, during which the cancer may grow or spread to regional lymph nodes. This again has a negative effect on prognosis and may require modifications to the treatment plan.[8] Alternatively, an improved prognosis can arise if on final pathology a tumor is found smaller than originally thought at the time of clinical staging or a clinically positive neck is revealed to have only an inflammatory enlarged node and a pathologically negative neck specimen.

CONSIDERATIONS FOR N STAGING

TNM clinical staging for head and neck cancer has undergone periodic revisions throughout its history. Although there have not been significant revisions to the nodal (N) staging system, there has been much discussion about the significance of the location of nodal disease, lymph node density, and the presence of ECE. Current nodal classification includes the size, multiplicity, and laterality of cervical metastasis (see **Table 1**).

Proposed changes designate *U* for upper neck lesions and *L* for lower neck lesions because distant metastasis rates vary depending on level of cervical metastases. The 5-year survival rate decreases with lower levels of metastatic nodes, from 37% for level I to 25% for level IV nodal involvement.[14] Lower levels of nodal disease also suggest a greater burden of metastatic disease, because the presence of level IV nodal disease is likely associated with multiple lesions in the neck.[15] Also, investigations have demonstrated an association between lymph node density and outcome. Lymph node density has been used to guide prognosis in breast, bladder, and gastrointestinal malignancies and has recently been applied to head and neck cancer to suggest prognostic value, specifically in oral cavity SCC.[16] Proponents for lymph node density argue that traditional pathologic N staging does not accurately reflect prognosis because it does not account for the total number of lymph nodes involved.[17–19] The lymph node density is defined by the total number of positive lymph nodes to the total number of lymph nodes within the dissection.[20] This system attempts to correct for pathologic understaging by incorporating the extent of nodal disease (total nodes involved) and the thoroughness of the surgery and pathologic evaluation (total nodes examined). Several studies have defined the ideal lymph node density threshold as less than or equal to 0.06, demonstrating an overall 5-year survival rate of 58% versus 26%.[19] However, 0.20 and 0.16 are also referenced within the literature, with similar poor outcomes associated with an increased lymph node density value.[19–23]

ECE and positive resection margins are 2 pathologic features that warrant the use of adjuvant chemotherapy and radiation therapy in advanced head and neck cancer.[18,24] Described in multiple studies, the presence of ECE in oral cavity cancer is an independent negative prognostic factor. Recently, Maxwell and colleagues[24] reported a 3-year disease-specific survival rate of 45% with ECE and 71% without the presence of ECE.[25,26] ECE is also associated with increased number of nodal metastasis, regional recurrences, and distant metastases.[24,27,28] ECE may not have as profound an influence on prognosis in oropharynx cancer, because no significant difference in survival was found in comparison to patients without ECE.[24]

SQUAMOUS CELL CARCINOMA

Head and neck cancer represents 4% of all cancers in the United States. Among head and neck cancers, SCC represents approximately 90% of all malignancies of the head and neck. SCC can be encountered at multiple sites within the head and neck, such as the oral cavity, skin, pharynx, paranasal sinuses, and salivary glands. Common among all locations is the sequence of metastasis, wherein most SCC travels first to the neck prior to distant metastasis. Tumor cells from the primary site find their way into the labyrinth of lymphatics that drain through a series of lymph nodes in the

neck. Conceptually acting as filters, lymph nodes trap cancer cells where they can often evade host defense mechanisms and proliferate. The detection of cancer within cervical nodes decreases curability by 50%.[3,4] The status of the neck should always be considered when formulating a treatment plan. Because of the critical significance of cervical metastasis, there exists a significant amount of literature on the risk factors for nodal spread in addition to techniques on the evaluation of the neck for cervical disease.

The general indications for surgical intervention in an N-positive neck include the presence of clinically enlarged nodes as identified on physical examination or by imaging. Surgical interrogation of the neck is also performed to identify and remove potentially involved lymph nodes as demonstrated by a lack of clinical evidence by means of physical examination or imaging. Intervention on a clinically negative (N0) neck is based on the likelihood of occult disease in the neck. Weiss and colleagues[29] deduced that treatment of the neck is warranted if the probability of occult cervical metastasis is greater than 20%, and this threshold has been the classic basis of treatment in N0 situations.

Studies on risk factors for metastatic cervical disease are ongoing. The following are commonly assessed features for the risk of developing cervical spread:

- Tumor location is a significant factor in determining the location and pattern of cervical spread. The oral cavity includes 8 subsites, each of which has its own tendencies for regional metastasis. For oral cavity cancers, the most common neck regions for cervical spread are levels I to III. Oropharynx, hypopharynx, and laryngeal cancers frequently travel to level II through level IV.[5,10,30]
- Evaluation of the contralateral neck is a strong consideration for oral cavity and oropharyngeal lesions presenting at or near the midline or extending across the midline, in addition to tumors greater than T3 size.[31,32] Koo and colleagues[31] reported that among patients with midline lesions and clinically evident ipsilateral neck disease, 36% harbored occult contralateral disease.
- Tumor size in conjunction with location help differentiate the risk of cervical disease. Oral cavity cancers staged as T2 and greater are generally indicated for neck dissection, because studies have estimated the rate of cervical spread as 14% with T1 tumors, 37% with T2, and 57% with T3/T4.[33] Furthermore, the relationship between tumor thickness

and occult cervical spread has been studied extensively. The threshold for neck dissection varies between institutions but typically ranges from 2 mm to 4 mm.[7,12,13,34] Studies have revealed that T1 and T2 SCCs of the oral tongue with a thickness greater than 4 mm were associated with a risk of neck disease, with an occult cervical metastasis rate of 30%.[12,13] The threshold for thickness varies with location, with lesions of the floor of mouth demonstrating a cervical metastasis rate of 33% in tumor thicknesses greater than 1.6 mm, with a significant increased cervical metastasis rate to 60% with thicknesses greater than 3.6 mm.[35] Maxillary lesions were reported to have a regional metastasis rate of 31.4% in lesions greater than T2.[36]

SALIVARY GLAND CANCERS

Salivary gland cancers of the head and neck account for 3% to 5% of all head and neck cancers.[37] As with other cancers, staging of the neck stems from a combination of physical examination and imaging. Defining features are the location of the primary tumor, size, and laterality.

Similar to SCC of the head and neck, the decision for surgical intervention of an N0 neck is based on the probability of a primary salivary tumor to metastasize to the neck lymphatics. In general, salivary malignancies metastasize much less frequently to cervical lymph nodes compared with SCC, but the presence of nodal disease as manifested by physical findings or imaging is an indication for a comprehensive neck dissection. In the setting of an N0 neck, indications for an elective neck dissection include an advanced primary tumor staging (>4 cm) or high-grade tumors (high-grade mucoepidermoid carcinoma, undifferentiated carcinoma, salivary duct carcinoma, and adenocarcinoma).[38,39] Overall, salivary gland cancers demonstrate an occult cervical metastasis range from 8% to 19%, although a recent study reported a rate of 39.5%.[40–42] Of the more common salivary gland tumors, adenoid cystic carcinoma (ACC) has a greater tendency for distant metastasis than for regional lymph node involvement. Unlike SCC, 33% to 50% of patients with ACC who develop distant metastasis do not present with regional disease.[43,44] Distant metastasis occurs in a majority of ACC patients, 22% to 60%.[45]

CARCINOMA OF UNKNOWN PRIMARY

Cervical metastasis in the absence of an identified primary tumor is termed, *carcinoma of unknown primary*. Approximately 2% to 9% of patients

make up this group of head and neck cancers.[46] The tonsillar fossa and base of tongue region are the most likely sites to harbor an occult primary cancer.[47] Presentation within the neck frequently involves levels II and III; bilateral adenopathy is present in approximately 10% of patients; and median nodal size has been reported as 5 cm.[48–50] Supraclavicular lymphadenopathy is less likely associated with head and neck cancer and is more often associated with a primary cancer below the clavicles.[46] **Figs. 2** and **3** illustrate a patient with a supraclavicular metastatic lymphadenopathy originating from a primary cancer within the lung.

After confirmation of a malignant diagnosis with a fine-needle aspiration biopsy, investigation to discover the primary tumor includes an evaluation under anesthesia and panendoscopy. Directed biopsies of high risk areas such as the base of tongue, tonsil, pyriform sinus and nasopharynx can be considered. A tonsillectomy is commonly recommended because up to 25% of primary occult tumors are located in this area. The use of transoral robotic surgery (TORS) to assist in the identification of an occult primary has demonstrated encouraging results. Preliminary results with TORS base of tongue resection show an increase in the overall detection rate for carcinoma of unknown primary.[51,52] Without clinical signs of tumor, imaging with MRI, CT, and PET has a detection rate of 20% to 25%.[47] Greatest detection rates

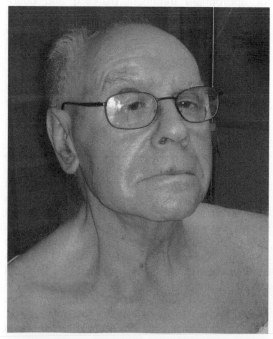

Fig. 2. Right supraclavicular metastatic SCC without other lymphadenopathy.

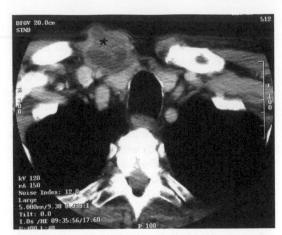

Fig. 3. Axial CT image shows a right supraclavicular metastasis with irregular borders and central lucency (*asterisk*). Primary SCC was later identified in the right lung.

are noted after the completion of physical examination, imaging and biopsies, approximating 40% to 65%.[47,51–53]

EVALUATION OF THE NECK FOR NODAL METASTASIS

The evaluation of the neck is an essential part of the management of head and neck cancer. The identification of cervical lymphadenopathy is a significant negative prognostic finding and allows for appropriate treatment planning and counseling. Multiple modalities of US, CT, MRI, and PET are currently used as part of the evaluation of the head and neck. Beginning with the physical examination, it has been assessed to demonstrate a sensitivity, specificity, and accuracy of 74%, 81%, and 77%, respectively.[54] The inaccuracy of the physical examination is improved by use of diagnostic imaging.

Ultrasound

The neck is ideal for US assessment due to the superficial nature of the underlying structures. This imaging modality is commonly used to assess cervical lymphadenopathy and is often combined to assist in fine-needle biopsy. It is common practice among head and neck units in Europe.[55] US is superior to physical examination and in multiple studies has a higher sensitivity in detecting nodal disease compared with conventional imaging.[56,57] Relative to CT, MRI, and PET imaging, US is readily available, cost effective, and noninvasive. In conjunction with fine-needle aspiration cytology, US imaging is highly specific for the evaluation of nodal metastases.[58]

Within the context of US examination of the neck, lymph nodes are normally identifiable in 4 anatomic locations: parotid, submandibular, upper cervical, and posterior triangle regions.[57] The presence of enlarged lymph nodes outside of these 4 regions should raise suspicion for a pathologic process. Node size is a distinguishing characteristic of nodal malignancy but only in association with additional features. The width of the node is considered the more specific dimension to assess and should not exceed 10 mm. Sensitivity and specificity at the threshold of 10 mm are 63% and 92%, respectively, for the detection of metastatic disease.[59] Moghaddam and colleagues[60] demonstrated that a 7-mm diameter cutoff corresponds to a sensitivity of 85% and 79%, respectively. In relation to the primary tumor, studies have been conducted to assess depth of invasion by US assessment. The accuracy of ultrasonic measurement between 3 mm and 15 mm demonstrated accuracy approximating 91%.[61,62]

The outline and shape of a normal lymph node should be that of a well-defined kidney bean (**Fig. 4**B). Irregular borders can represent metastatic disease in 84.6% of nodes and may also suggest the presence of extracapsular spread (**Fig. 4**F).[63] With a width-to-length ratio greater than 0.5, suggesting a spherical shape, a node is highly suspicious for metastatic disease (**Fig. 4**C, D).[55] Normal submandibular, submental, and parotid lymph nodes can be rounded; hence, shape should not be used as an independent marker for malignancy.[55,57,60]

Although benign, reactive and most metastatic nodes are hypoechoic, with cortical thickening, the presence of a hyperechoic cervical lymph node, or calcification indicative of a thyroid cancer.[64,65]

The vascular pattern of lymph nodes can be readily assessed with color and Doppler ultrasonography. Normal blood flow within a lymph node occurs in a central or hilar distribution (see **Fig. 4**A). Malignant nodes feature a peripheral or mixed hilar and peripheral vascular pattern (see **Fig. 4**E). The addition of microbubble intravenous contrast can enhance the resolution between vascular patterns and echogenic areas. Contrast-enhanced US is described as having a sensitivity of 92%, specificity of 93%, and accuracy of 92.8% for the detection of metastatic disease within lymph nodes.[66]

CT and MRI Evaluation of the Neck

CT and MRI are an integral part of the preoperative work-up and post-therapeutic surveillance because

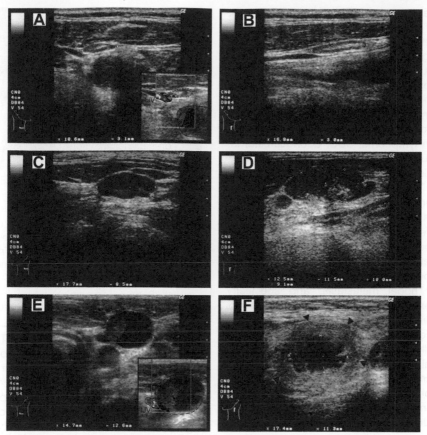

Fig. 4. Example of US findings in cervical lymph nodes. (*A*) Axial view of a normal lymph node. Note the uniform echogenic parenchyma, smooth borders, and oval shape. (*Inset*) Duplex view, lymph node identified by dashed line with hilar vascular pattern. CA, carotid artery; IJV, internal jugular vein. (*B*) Longitudinal view of a normal lymph node. (*C*) Metastatic disease in a lymph node. Note the heterogenous parenchymal echotexture and surface irregularity. (*D*) Metastatic disease in 2 lymph nodes with spherical form and matting. (*E*) Metastatic disease in lymph node with intranodal cystic necrosis. (*Inset*) Duplex view, aberrant intranodal vessels. (*F*) Lymph node metastasis with intranodal cystic necrosis, lack of nodal borders, and diffuse extracapsular infiltration (*arrowheads*). (*From* Roper B, Nuse N, Busch R, et al. Tissue characterization of locoregionally advanced head-and-neck squamous cell carcinoma [HNSCC] using quantified ultrasonography: a prospective phase II study on prognostic relevance. Radiother Oncol 2007;85:48.)

the course of patients with head and neck cancer is profoundly affected by the presence of cervical metastasis. Regardless of the site of the primary origin of an SCC, the presence of a single metastatic lymph node reduces the survival by 50%, the presence of bilateral cervical metastasis reduces the survival by another 50%, and the existence of extranodal disease and/or fixed nodes further reduces prognosis.[3,4] In addition to assessment of the neck for nodal disease, the high-quality cross-sectional imaging afforded by CT and MRI enables surgeons to assess the resectability of the primary tumor as well as that of the cervical metastases. The presence of carotid encasement or fixation of the tumor to the skull base or prevertebral fascia/space obviates a surgical option.

Specific features are examined to assess for the presence of metastatic disease in cross-sectional imaging modalities, such as CT, MRI, and US.[67] These features include nodal size, location, contour, calcifications, and central necrosis.[67] Lymph nodes greater than 1 cm are generally considered abnormal, with 88% sensitivity and 39% specificity for metastatic disease.[67,68] With lymph nodes in level I and level IIa, an increase in diameter is tolerated to 1.5 cm because they are more likely affected by benign hyperplasia than other nodal groups.[68] Retropharyngeal nodes that exceed 0.8 cm carry a high risk of metastatic disease. These are more common in thyroid and nasopharyngeal cancers.[67] Nodes less than 1 cm in size can still harbor metastasis and should be carefully evaluated for other abnormal features, particularly if the node is located within a predicted drainage pattern.

The changes in contour of malignant cervical nodes result from internal alterations as microscopic tumor deposits replace the normal fatty hila producing features, such as calcifications, necrosis, enhancement, and cystic changes.[68] Along with thyroid cancers, calcifications may present in patients with lymphoma, SCC, adenocarcinoma, and tuberculosis, although less commonly.[69] Necrotic nodes appear on CT with focal hypoattenuation or on T2 MRI with hyperintensity and irregular peripheral enhancement (**Figs. 5** and **6**).[68] The necrosis is located in the center of the lymph node and reflects an obstruction of lymphatic flow by tumor cells, fibrous tissue, and edema. The combination of a lymph node with nodal necrosis and the presence of a primary tumor are highly specific for nodal metastasis, and specificity approximates 100%.[70] Cystic nodes are suggestive for a primary oropharyngeal SCC or papillary thyroid cancer. On MRI or CT, cystic nodes appear as a thin-walled fluid collection and can present as a large nodal lesion despite originating from small or occult primary cancers. Cystic nodes can also be misinterpreted as branchial cleft cysts; hence, a comprehensive survey should be completed as part of a patient's work-up (**Fig. 7**).

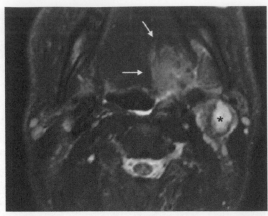

Fig. 6. Axial T2 MRI with enhancement of SCC of the base of tongue (*arrows*). *Asterisk* denotes area of central necrotic enlarged lymph nodes. (*From* Beil CM, Keberle M. Oral and oropharyngeal tumors. Eur J Radiol 2008;66:448.)

PET/CT

Fludeoxyglucose F 18–enhanced PET is an imaging modality that evaluates for metabolically active tissue, such as cancer, and is used for staging and surveillance in head and neck cancer. Although PET can be vulnerable to false-positive and false-negative results, the sensitivity of PET imaging approaches 85% and specificity of 86%.[71] Inflammation and muscular activity can confound the results of PET. The negative and positive predictive values of PET for detecting residual and recurrent head and neck cancer are 75% and 95%, respectively.[72] Current techniques combine PET with an anatomic scan, such as CT or MRI, to allow for accurate localization of suspected

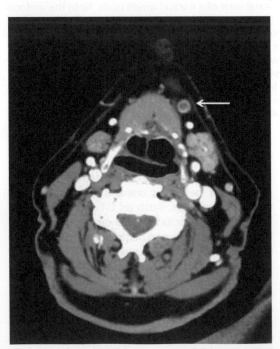

Fig. 5. Axial CT image at the level of the submandibular gland. Left level Ib lymph node with metastatic disease. Note the round lymph node and hypoattenuation indicating intranodal necrosis (*arrow*).

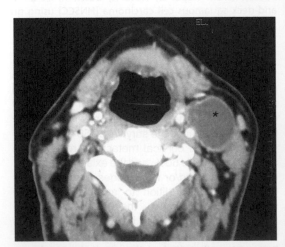

Fig. 7. Axial CT image of an isolated cystic metastasis (*asterisk*) from an occult lesion in the ipsilateral tonsil. The lesion is deceptively similar to a second branchial cleft cyst.

nodal disease and distant metastasis. Detection for disease less than 4 to 5 mm is limited.[73] In the pretreatment setting, the use of PET/CT or MRI can provide prognostic value based on the intensity of the primary lesion (**Fig. 8**). The unit of measurement is the subjective uptake value (SUV); values greater than 2.5 to 3.5 SUV are considered abnormal.[74] SUV thresholds for a poor prognosis are reported to range between 5 and 10 SUV.[75–77] Average value for a head and neck cancer primary approximates 8 SUV.[78] Studies have reviewed the prognostic value in relation to intensity of SUV with the consensus demonstrating an association between an increase in SUV with decrease in survival.[73,79] As a continuous variable, an increased relative risk of death of 14% for each 1-unit increase in SUV has been described.[80] Studies also suggest an association between elevated SUV and incidence of ECE and higher rates of locoregional recurrence.[76,81]

Sentinel Lymph Node Biopsy

Adjunctive procedures that assist in staging include sentinel lymph node biopsy (SNB). Although patients undergo general anesthesia for the resection of the primary and SNB, the extent of the neck dissection is limited to the area of the sentinel node. It is indicated for N0 patients who fall under the risk of occult metastasis and present with a T1 or T2 primary oral cavity. Through sentinel node biopsy, the initial lymph node draining a particular tumor area, the sentinel node, is identified and excised to assess for the presence of metastasis. Serial sectioning and immunohistochemistry to detect the presence of metastasis

have demonstrated results with high sensitivity and specificity.[82,83] The likelihood of a missed occult metastasis due to sampling error is slim with a negative predictive value of 89% to 96%.[82] Inherent to this procedure is the possibility of upward stage migration.

Neck Evaluation During Post-therapeutic Surveillance

The onset of new pain has been shown to be the first symptom and an independent factor of recurrent head and neck cancer within the first year of surveillance.[84] Patients who do not present with pain or other overt signs or symptoms rely on imaging to monitor for the features of recurrence. There are no defined guidelines for post-therapeutic imaging; however, contemporary trends suggest that it begin 3 to 6 months after therapy completion.[72,85] Post-surgery and adjuvant therapy, the assessment of the head and neck can be challenging. The effects of ablative and reconstructive surgery, radiation, and chemotherapy can drastically alter the landscape of normal anatomy. Effective treatment depends on the ability to differentiate between benign and malignant changes.

Non-neoplastic soft tissue changes after radiation therapy occur within 2 weeks of therapy and have been described to transition from an acute inflammatory reaction to the development of fibrosis. On imaging, the changes identified on CT and MRI manifest as thickening of the skin and platysma muscle, reticulation of the subcutaneous and deep tissue fat layers, retropharyngeal space edema and effusion, increased enhancement of

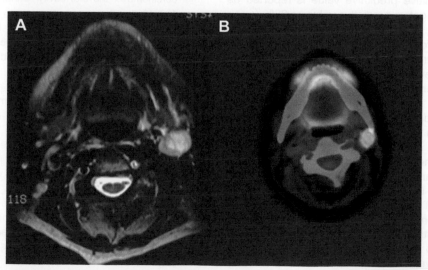

Fig. 8. (*A*) Axial T2 MRI with enhancement of a left metastatic level II lymphadenopathy. (*B*) Axial CT/PET demonstrating enhancement of the left level II metastatic node, with an SUV of 22.4.

the major salivary glands, thickening and enhancement of the mucsoa of the upper aerodigestive tract, and increased density and stranding in paralaryngeal fat.[86,87] These changes are dependent on the target radiation field and dosage. Intensity-modulated radiation therapy attempts to reduce the collateral radiation field by targeting the area of interest via multiple radiation ports. Changes secondary to radiation peak within the first few months of completing radiotherapy but may persist for 12 to 18 months.[86,88]

A comparison with baseline imaging provides valuable information on the interpretation of all forms of surveillance imaging. Basic principles assist in the detection of recurrent or persistent disease with the understanding that a new or enlarging neck mass should be considered recurrence until proved otherwise. A common location for treatment failure is within the operative bed or along surgical margins.[88] Recurrent tumors present with features similar to the development of a primary tumor or cervical lymphadenopathy, as discussed previously. CT has a high sensitivity and moderate specificity for differentiating recurrent tumor from post-treatment changes.[89,90] The limitation of CT in discerning between fibrotic tissues versus recurrent tumor can be resolved with the use of MRI. T2-weighted MRI is able to assess an abnormal mass to differentiate between tumor and dense fibrous tissue.[88,91]

PET imaging in post-therapeutic surveillance has increased the ability to detect the presence of recurrent disease.[92] Sensitivity and specificity of PET in detecting residual and recurrent head and neck cancer are 94% and 82%, respectively.[72] Positive predictive value is reported as 75% and negative predictive value as 95%.[72]

Generally, post-therapeutic surveillance patients are followed clinically for the first 8 to 12 weeks, unless clinical findings suggest a need for further evaluation with CT and/or MRI scan. PET is deferred during the first 8 to 12 weeks; this range varies depending on institution, because radiation and postsurgical changes can lead to high false-positive results. Studies report a predictive accuracy of PET/CT scans of 100% when obtained later than 8 weeks versus 76.5% between 4 and 8 weeks.[93,94] After this period, patients may undergo imaging with CT, MRI, or another PET every 3 to 6 months depending on physician preference. Tumor recurrence is most frequent within the first 3 years after therapy. Although no defined guidelines exist on the duration of surveillance, most patients are routinely followed for 3 to 5 years.[92,95,96] Unfortunately, despite the identification of disease prior to overt

clinical signs of recurrence, the mortality for salvage therapy remains high.[97]

REFERENCES

1. Jemal A, Siegel R, Xu J, et al. Cancer statistics, 2010. CA Cancer J Clin 2010;60(5):277–300.
2. Greenlee RT, Murray T, Bolden S, et al. Cancer statistics, 2000. CA Cancer J Clin 2010;50(1):7–33.
3. Leemans CR, Tiwari R, Nauta JJ, et al. Regional lymph node involvement and its significance in the development of distant metastases in head and neck carcinoma. Cancer 1993;71(2):452–6.
4. Leemans CR, Tiwari R, Nauta JJ, et al. Recurrence at the primary site in head and neck cancer and the significance of neck lymph node metastases as a prognostic factor. Cancer 1994;73(1):187–90.
5. Shah JP. Patterns of cervical lymph node metastasis from squamous carcinomas of the upper aerodigestive tract. Am J Surg 1990;160(4):405–9.
6. Lindberg R. Distribution of cervical lymph node metastases from squamous cell carcinoma of the upper respiratory and digestive tracts. Cancer 1972;29(6):1446–9.
7. Ord RA. Surgical management of the N0 neck in early stage T1-2 oral cancer; a personal perspective of early and late impalpable disease. Oral Maxillofac Surg 2012;16(2):181–8.
8. Sobin LH. TNM: evolution and relation to other prognostic factors. Semin Surg Oncol 2003;21(1):3–7.
9. Edge SB, Byrd DR, Compton CC, et al, editors. AJCC cancer staging manual. 7th edition. Springer Science and Business Media; 2010.
10. Shah JP, Candela FC, Poddar AK. The patterns of cervical lymph node metastases from squamous carcinoma of the oral cavity. Cancer 1990;66(1):109–13.
11. Yuen AP, Wei WI, Wong YM, et al. Elective neck dissection versus observation in the treatment of early oral tongue carcinoma. Head Neck 1997;19(7):583–8.
12. Kligerman J, Lima RA, Soares JR, et al. Supraomohyoid neck dissection in the treatment of T1/T2 squamous cell carcinoma of oral cavity. Am J Surg 1994;168(5):391–4.
13. Fakih AR, Rao RS, Borges AM, et al. Elective versus therapeutic neck dissection in early carcinoma of the oral tongue. Am J Surg 1989;158(4):309–13.
14. Jones AS, Roland NJ, Field JK, et al. The level of cervical lymph node metastases: their prognostic relevance and relationship with head and neck squamous carcinoma primary sites. Clin Otolaryngol Allied Sci 1994;19(1):63–9.
15. Dias FL, Lima RA, Kligerman J, et al. Relevance of skip metastases for squamous cell carcinoma of

the oral tongue and the floor of the mouth. Otolaryngol Head Neck Surg 2006;134(3):460–5.

16. van der Wal BC, Butzelaar RM, van der Meij S, et al. Axillary lymph node ratio and total number of removed lymph nodes: predictors of survival in stage I and II breast cancer. Eur J Surg Oncol 2002;28(5):481–9.

17. Shingaki S, Takada M, Sasai K, et al. Impact of lymph node metastasis on the pattern of failure and survival in oral carcinomas. Am J Surg 2003; 185(3):278–84.

18. Bernier J, Cooper JS, Pajak TF, et al. Defining risk levels in locally advanced head and neck cancers: a comparative analysis of concurrent postoperative radiation plus chemotherapy trials of the EORTC (#22931) and RTOG (# 9501). Head Neck 2005; 27(10):843–50.

19. Gil Z, Carlson DL, Boyle JO, et al. Lymph node density is a significant predictor of outcome in patients with oral cancer. Cancer 2009;115(24): 5700–10.

20. Rudra S, Spiotto MT, Witt ME, et al. Lymph node density - Prognostic value in head and neck cancer. Head Neck 2014;36(2):266–72.

21. Ebrahimi A, Clark JR, Zhang WJ, et al. Lymph node ratio as an independent prognostic factor in oral squamous cell carcinoma. Head Neck 2011; 33(9):1245–51.

22. Kim SY, Nam SY, Choi SH, et al. Prognostic value of lymph node density in node-positive patients with oral squamous cell carcinoma. Ann Surg Oncol 2011;18(8):2310–7.

23. Liao CT, Hsueh C, Lee LY, et al. Neck dissection field and lymph node density predict prognosis in patients with oral cavity cancer and pathological node metastases treated with adjuvant therapy. Oral Oncol 2012;48(4):329–36.

24. Maxwell JH, Ferris RL, Gooding W, et al. Extracapsular spread in head and neck carcinoma: impact of site and human papillomavirus status. Cancer 2013;119(18):3302–8.

25. Shaw RJ, Lowe D, Woolgar JA, et al. Extracapsular spread in oral squamous cell carcinoma. Head Neck 2010;32(6):714–22.

26. Myers JN, Greenberg JS, Mo V, et al. Extracapsular spread. A significant predictor of treatment failure in patients with squamous cell carcinoma of the tongue. Cancer 2001;92(12):3030–6.

27. Alvi A, Johnson JT. Development of distant metastasis after treatment of advanced-stage head and neck cancer. Head Neck 1997;19(6):500–5.

28. Greenberg JS, Fowler R, Gomez J, et al. Extent of extracapsular spread: a critical prognosticator in oral tongue cancer. Cancer 2003;97(6): 1464–70.

29. Weiss MH, Harrison LB, Isaacs RS. Use of decision analysis in planning a management strategy for the stage N0 neck. Arch Otolaryngol Head Neck Surg 1994;120(7):699–702.

30. Candela FC, Kothari K, Shah JP. Patterns of cervical node metastases from squamous carcinoma of the oropharynx and hypopharynx. Head Neck 1990;12(3):197–203.

31. Koo BS, Lim YC, Lee JS, et al. Management of contralateral N0 neck in oral cavity squamous cell carcinoma. Head Neck 2006;28(10):896–901.

32. Lim YC, Lee SY, Lim JY, et al. Management of contralateral N0 neck in tonsillar squamous cell carcinoma. Laryngoscope 2005;115(9):1672–5.

33. Tytor M, Olofsson J. Prognostic factors in oral cavity carcinomas. Acta Otolaryngol Suppl 1992;492: 75–8.

34. Spiro RH, Huvos AG, Wong GY, et al. Predictive value of tumor thickness in squamous carcinoma confined to the tongue and floor of the mouth. Am J Surg 1986;152(4):345–50.

35. Mohit-Tabatabai MA, Sobel HJ, Rush BF, et al. Relation of thickness of floor of mouth stage I and II cancers to regional metastasis. Am J Surg 1986;152(4):351–3.

36. Montes DM, Carlson ER, Fernandes R, et al. Oral maxillary squamous carcinoma: an indication for neck dissection in the clinically negative neck. Head Neck 2011;33(11):1581–5.

37. Spiro RH. Salivary neoplasms: overview of a 35-year experience with 2,807 patients. Head Neck Surg 1986;8(3):177–84.

38. Bell RB, Dierks EJ, Homer L, et al. Management and outcome of patients with malignant salivary gland tumors. J Oral Maxillofac Surg 2005;63(7): 917–28.

39. Adelstein DJ, Koyfman SA, El-Naggar AK, et al. Biology and management of salivary gland cancers. Semin Radiat Oncol 2012;22(3):245–53.

40. Armstrong JG, Harrison LB, Thaler HT, et al. The indications for elective treatment of the neck in cancer of the major salivary glands. Cancer 1992; 69(3):615–9.

41. Medina JE. Neck dissection in the treatment of cancer of major salivary glands. Otolaryngol Clin North Am 1998;31(5):815–22.

42. Nobis CP, Rohleder NH, Wolff KD, et al. Head and Neck Salivary Gland Carcinomas-Elective Neck Dissection, Yes or No? J Oral Maxillofac Surg 2014;72(1):205–10.

43. Rapidis AD, Givalos N, Gakiopoulou H, et al. Adenoid cystic carcinoma of the head and neck. Clinicopathological analysis of 23 patients and review of the literature. Oral Oncol 2005;41(3):328–35.

44. Spiro RH. Distant metastasis in adenoid cystic carcinoma of salivary origin. Am J Surg 1997;174(5): 495–8.

45. Sung MW, Kim KH, Kim JW, et al. Clinicopathologic predictors and impact of distant metastasis from

adenoid cystic carcinoma of the head and neck. Arch Otolaryngol Head Neck Surg 2003;129(11): 1193–7.

46. Million RR, Cassisi NJ, Mancuso AA. Management of head and neck cancer: a multidisciplinary approach. 2nd edition. Philadelphia: Lippincott; 1994. p. 311–21.

47. Cianchetti M, Mancuso AA, Amdur RJ, et al. Diagnostic evaluation of squamous cell carcinoma metastatic to cervical lymph nodes from an unknown head and neck primary site. Laryngoscope 2009; 119(12):2348–54.

48. Strojan P, Anicin A. Combined surgery and postoperative radiotherapy for cervical lymph node metastases from an unknown primary tumour. Radiother Oncol 1998;49(1):33–40.

49. Erkal HS, Mendenhall WM, Amdur RJ, et al. Squamous cell carcinomas metastatic to cervical lymph nodes from an unknown head-and-neck mucosal site treated with radiation therapy alone or in combination with neck dissection. Int J Radiat Oncol Biol Phys 2001;50(1):55–63.

50. Jereczek-Fossa BA, Jassem J, Orecchia R. Cervical lymph node metastases of squamous cell carcinoma from an unknown primary. Cancer Treat Rev 2004;30(2):153–64.

51. Abuzeid WM, Bradford CR, Divi V. Transoral robotic biopsy of the tongue base: a novel paradigm in the evaluation of unknown primary tumors of the head and neck. Head Neck 2013;35(4):E126–30.

52. Mehta V, Johnson P, Tassler A, et al. A new paradigm for the diagnosis and management of unknown primary tumors of the head and neck: a role for transoral robotic surgery. Laryngoscope 2013;123(1):146–51.

53. Mendenhall WM, Mancuso AA, Parsons JT, et al. Diagnostic evaluation of squamous cell carcinoma metastatic to cervical lymph nodes from an unknown head and neck primary site. Head Neck 1998;20(8): 739–44.

54. Merritt RM, Williams MF, James TH, et al. Detection of cervical metastasis. A meta-analysis comparing computed tomography with physical examination. Arch Otolaryngol Head Neck Surg 1997;123(2): 149–52.

55. Oeppen RS, Gibson D, Brennan PA. An update on the use of ultrasound imaging in oral and maxillofacial surgery. Br J Oral Maxillofac Surg 2010;48(6): 412–8.

56. Jeong HS, Baek CH, Son YI, et al. Use of integrated 18F-FDG PET/CT to improve the accuracy of initial cervical nodal evaluation in patients with head and neck squamous cell carcinoma. Head Neck 2007;29(3):203–10.

57. Giacomini CP, Jeffrey RB, Shin LK. Ultrasonographic evaluation of malignant and normal cervical lymph nodes. Semin Ultrasound CT MR 2013; 34(3):236–47.

58. van den Brekel MW, Castelijns JA, Stel HV, et al. Occult metastatic neck disease: detection with US and US-guided fine-needle aspiration cytology. Radiology 1991;180(2):457–61.

59. van den Brekel MW, Pameijer FA, Koops W, et al. Computed tomography for the detection of neck node metastases in melanoma patients. Eur J Surg Oncol 1998;24(1):51–4.

60. Imani Moghaddam M, Davachi B, Mostaan LV, et al. Evaluation of the sonographic features of metastatic cervical lymph nodes in patients with head and neck malignancy. J Craniofac Surg 2011; 22(6):2179–84.

61. Yuen AP, Ng RW, Lam PK, et al. Preoperative measurement of tumor thickness of oral tongue carcinoma with intraoral ultrasonography. Head Neck 2008;30(2):230–4.

62. Kodama M, Khanal A, Habu M, et al. Ultrasonography for intraoperative determination of tumor thickness and resection margin in tongue carcinomas. J Oral Maxillofac Surg 2010;68(8):1746–52.

63. Toriyabe Y, Nishimura T, Kita S, et al. Differentiation between benign and metastatic cervical lymph nodes with ultrasound. Clin Radiol 1997;52(12): 927–32.

64. Rosario PW, de Faria S, Bicalho L, et al. Ultrasonographic differentiation between metastatic and benign lymph nodes in patients with papillary thyroid carcinoma. J Ultrasound Med 2005;24(10): 1385–9.

65. Chan JM, Shin LK, Jeffrey RB. Ultrasonography of abnormal neck lymph nodes. Ultrasound Q 2007; 23(1):47–54.

66. Rubaltelli L, Khadivi Y, Tregnaghi A, et al. Evaluation of lymph node perfusion using continuous mode harmonic ultrasonography with a second-generation contrast agent. J Ultrasound Med 2004;23(6):829–36.

67. Som PM. Detection of metastasis in cervical lymph nodes: CT and MR criteria and differential diagnosis. AJR Am J Roentgenol 1992;158(5):961–9.

68. Hoang JK, Vanka J, Ludwig BJ, et al. Evaluation of cervical lymph nodes in head and neck cancer with CT and MRI: tips, traps, and a systematic approach. AJR Am J Roentgenol 2013;200(1):W17–25.

69. Eisenkraft BL, Som PM. The spectrum of benign and malignant etiologies of cervical node calcification. AJR Am J Roentgenol 1999;172(5):1433–7.

70. Kaji AV, Mohuchy T, Swartz JD. Imaging of cervical lymphadenopathy. Semin Ultrasound CT MR 1997; 18(3):220–49.

71. Kyzas PA, Evangelou E, Denaxa-Kyza D, et al. 18F-fluorodeoxyglucose positron emission tomography to evaluate cervical node metastases in patients with head and neck squamous cell carcinoma: a meta-analysis. J Natl Cancer Inst 2008;100(10): 712–20.

72. Al-Ibraheem A, Buck A, Krause BJ, et al. Clinical Applications of FDG PET and PET/CT in Head and Neck Cancer. J Oncol 2009;2009:208725.

73. Schoder H, Carlson DL, Kraus DH, et al. 18F-FDG PET/CT for detecting nodal metastases in patients with oral cancer staged N0 by clinical examination and CT/MRI. J Nucl Med 2006;47(5):755–62.

74. Schoder H, Gonen M. Screening for cancer with PET and PET/CT: potential and limitations. J Nucl Med 2007;48(Suppl 1):4S–18S.

75. Kim SY, Roh JL, Kim JS, et al. Utility of FDG PET in patients with squamous cell carcinomas of the oral cavity. Eur J Surg Oncol 2008;34(2):208–15.

76. Schwartz DL, Rajendran J, Yueh B, et al. FDG-PET prediction of head and neck squamous cell cancer outcomes. Arch Otolaryngol Head Neck Surg 2004;130(12):1361–7.

77. Querellou S, Abgral R, Le Roux PY, et al. Prognostic value of fluorine-18 fluorodeoxyglucose positron-emission tomography imaging in patients with head and neck squamous cell carcinoma. Head Neck 2012;34(4):462–8.

78. Kubicek GJ, Champ C, Fogh S, et al. FDG-PET staging and importance of lymph node SUV in head and neck cancer. Head Neck Oncol 2010;2:19.

79. Nakajo M, Nakajo M, Kajiya Y, et al. FDG PET/CT and diffusion-weighted imaging of head and neck squamous cell carcinoma: comparison of prognostic significance between primary tumor standardized uptake value and apparent diffusion coefficient. Cancer Treat Rev 2012;37(5):475–80.

80. Wong RJ. Current status of FDG-PET for head and neck cancer. J Surg Oncol 2008;97(8):649–52.

81. Joo YH, Yoo IR, Cho KJ, et al. Extracapsular spread and FDG PET/CT correlations in oral squamous cell carcinoma. Int J Oral Maxillofac Surg 2013;42(2):158–63.

82. Broglie MA, Haile SR, Stoeckli SJ. Long-term experience in sentinel node biopsy for early oral and oropharyngeal squamous cell carcinoma. Ann Surg Oncol 2011;18(10):2732–8.

83. Civantos FJ, Zitsch RP, Schuller DE, et al. Sentinel lymph node biopsy accurately stages the regional lymph nodes for T1-T2 oral squamous cell carcinomas: results of a prospective multi-institutional trial. J Clin Oncol 2010;28(8):1395–400.

84. Scharpf J, Karnell LH, Christensen AJ, et al. The role of pain in head and neck cancer recurrence and survivorship. Arch Otolaryngol Head Neck Surg 2009;135(8):789–94.

85. Hermans R. Posttreatment imaging in head and neck cancer. Eur J Radiol 2008;66(3):501–11.

86. Mukherji SK, Mancuso AA, Kotzur IM, et al. Radiologic appearance of the irradiated larynx. Part I. Expected changes. Radiology 1994;193(1):141–8.

87. Hermans R. Post-treatment imaging of head and neck cancer. Cancer Imaging 2004;4(Spec No A):S6–15.

88. Offiah C, Hall E. Post-treatment imaging appearances in head and neck cancer patients. Clin Radiol 2011;66(1):13–24.

89. Lell M, Baum U, Greess H, et al. Head and neck tumors: imaging recurrent tumor and post-therapeutic changes with CT and MRI. Eur J Radiol 2000;33(3):239–47.

90. Lapela M, Eigtved A, Jyrkkio S, et al. Experience in qualitative and quantitative FDG PET in follow-up of patients with suspected recurrence from head and neck cancer. Eur J Cancer 2000; 36(7):858–67.

91. Hudgins PA. Flap reconstruction in the head and neck: expected appearance, complications, and recurrent disease. Eur J Radiol 2002;44(2):130–8.

92. Dunsky KA, Wehrmann DJ, Osman MM, et al. PET-CT and the detection of the asymptomatic recurrence or second primary lesions in the treated head and neck cancer patient. Laryngoscope 2013;123(9):2161–4.

93. Zhang I, Branstetter BF, Beswick DM, et al. The benefit of early PET/CT surveillance in HPV-associated head and neck squamous cell carcinoma. Arch Otolaryngol Head Neck Surg 2011; 137(11):1106–11.

94. Gourin CG, Williams HT, Seabolt WN, et al. Utility of positron emission tomography-computed tomography in identification of residual nodal disease after chemoradiation for advanced head and neck cancer. Laryngoscope 2006;116(5):705–10.

95. Ord RA, Kolokythas A, Reynolds MA. Surgical salvage for local and regional recurrence in oral cancer. J Oral Maxillofac Surg 2006;64(9):1409–14.

96. Liu G, Dierks EJ, Bell RB, et al. Post-therapeutic surveillance schedule for oral cancer: is there agreement? Oral Maxillofac Surg 2012;16(4): 327–40.

97. Ho AS, Tsao GJ, Chen FW, et al. Impact of positron emission tomography/computed tomography surveillance at 12 and 24 months for detecting head and neck cancer recurrence. Cancer 2013; 119(7):1349–56.

Update in Radiation Therapy for Oral and Maxillofacial Tumors and Dose Mapping

Ivan L. Kessel, MD[a],*, Angel Blanco, MD[b]

KEYWORDS

• Head and neck cancer • Radiation therapy • Intensity modulated radiation therapy (IMRT)

KEY POINTS

- Radiation therapy is an important modality in the treatment of head and neck cancers. High doses of radiation therapy are required to control these cancers.
- Normal tissues in the head and neck, adjacent to the primary tumors and draining lymph nodes, can experience severe toxicity from high doses of radiation therapy. The side effects of these toxicities can significantly affect important functions and quality of life for long-term survivors.
- Advances in the planning and delivery of radiation therapy, including intensity modulated radiation therapy, have resulted in significant sparing of normal tissues while adequately covering the target areas.

INTRODUCTION

Radiation therapy (RT) is an important treatment modality for most head and neck cancers. For many tumor sites, RT yields better functional outcomes than surgery and thus is often the preferred treatment for localized disease. For locoregionally advanced disease, RT is often used as adjuvant after surgery or (in combination with chemotherapy) either before surgery or as definitive organ-preserving treatment.

Ionizing radiation has its biologic effects by primarily causing DNA damage and loss of cellular reproductive ability. Some cells die rapidly through apoptosis (interphase death). Most cells, however, do not demonstrate evidence of damage until mitosis occurs (mitotic cell death). In fact, cell death may only occur after several cell divisions. The probability of cell death depends on the dose of radiation that the cell is exposed to. For DNA damage to be lethal to cells, the injury must be irreparable. Cells are able to repair sublethal damage, but the rate of repair differs in different tissues. By dividing the treatment into multiple fractions, a supralethal dose of radiation can be delivered to the tumor while allowing sparing of adjacent normal tissues, where the repair of sublethal damage may be more rapid or efficient. The best way of limiting the risk of damage to normal tissue, however, is to reduce the dose of radiation to that tissue.

Radiation can be administered by an external beam source or by brachytherapy (using either interstitial implants or intracavitary techniques). The choice of technique depends on the site of the tumor and the goal of therapy, and the available experience, skill, and technology. Most head and neck cancers are treated with external beam RT. The most commonly used forms of ionizing radiation are high-energy photons (ie, radiograph) and electrons, produced by linear accelerators. Photons with energies in the 4- to 6-MV range typically are used. The maximum tissue dose from these beams occurs several millimeters under the surface, resulting in an important

[a] Department of Radiation Oncology, University of Texas Medical Branch, 301 University Boulevard, Galveston, TX 77555, USA; [b] Memorial Hermann Hospital, 6400 Fannin Street, Houston, TX 77030, USA
* Corresponding author.
E-mail address: ilkessel@utmb.edu

Oral Maxillofacial Surg Clin N Am 26 (2014) 223–229
http://dx.doi.org/10.1016/j.coms.2014.01.008
1042-3699/14/$ – see front matter © 2014 Elsevier Inc. All rights reserved.

skin-sparing effect. To treat superficial lesions, a material with similar density to tissue ("bolus") can be placed directly overlying the lesion. The bolus can thus be designed to ensure that the maximum dose of absorbed radiation occurs on the skin surface. Electron beam therapy, with energies between 5 and 22 MV available on most linear accelerators, is used for superficial lesions. The dose beyond the treatment volume decreases much more rapidly with electrons than with photons. This feature may be exploited when there are critical structures located deep to the target volume. For example, electron beam therapy may be used to treat the posterior neck while sparing the spinal cord after maximum safe doses to the spinal cord have been given using photons. The use of neutrons and heavy charged particles, such as protons or carbon ions, remains investigational, although proton beam facilities are becoming more widely available. Although there are theoretical dosimetric advantages of proton beam therapy, sparing tissue located behind the target volume, there are no clinical trials comparing photon versus proton beam therapy in head and neck cancer to validate its routine use.

The techniques for planning and delivery of external beam RT for head and neck cancers have advanced dramatically, corresponding to the availability of increasingly powerful computer processors to make use of sophisticated 3-dimensional (3D) dose modeling programs routine. Advances in imaging give increased accuracy in localizing the tumors, and involve lymph nodes, as targets for RT. The treatment planning process involves the creation of target volumes, based on areas of known disease, or high risk of involvement to treat with an effective dose of radiation while limiting the exposure of adjacent normal structures, using either 3D conformal RT or intensity-modulated radiotherapy (IMRT). To ensure accuracy, a treatment planning computed tomographic (CT) scan is performed before therapy with the patient immobilized in the same position as will be used for treatments. The target volumes are outlined on this scan, as well as those normal structures that need to be spared from excess irradiation. Using 3D reconstruction of images, the spatial relationship of the target volumes to these normal anatomic structures is demonstrated. Other imaging techniques, including magnetic resonance imaging and positron emission tomography, may also be integrated in delineating soft tissue and tumor anatomy. Software manipulations allow these additional image sets to be fused with the planning CT to permit more accurate delineation of the target (tumor and involved lymph nodes) and of avoidance structures.

During treatment, the setup is verified by comparing bony structures on the planning CT scan with radiographs taken on the treatment linear accelerator. Megavoltage radiographs (portal films) are often used to verify the patient's position and the position of the radiation fields. Many facilities also have onboard kilovoltage radiograph imaging and/or cone-beam CT scanning capabilities incorporated into their linear accelerators to enable more precise image-guided patient localization before each treatment.

IMRT is a more sophisticated form of 3D conformal RT. IMRT uses multiple nonhomogeneous radiation beam intensities to maximize the delivery of radiation to the planned treatment volume while minimizing irradiation of normal tissue outside the target volumes. Inverse planning techniques are used, whereby the desired objectives for minimum dose to targets and maximum acceptable dose to avoidance structures are specified, and by working through multiple iterations of possible solutions, the treatment planning computer program tries to generate an optimal solution. IMRT is indicated for the treatment of most head and neck cancers (excluding early stage vocal cord cancer), requires additional time for planning computation and quality assurance verification, and results in the exposure of larger volumes of normal tissues to low doses of radiation.[1] A major advantage of IMRT in head and neck cancer is that it can reduce side effects (especially xerostomia) primarily by avoiding irradiation of the parotids. Parotid sparing has been shown in multiple studies to be associated with salivary function preservation and better recovery of saliva output. The benefit of IMRT in preventing xerostomia was also confirmed in the Parotid-sparing Intensity Modulated versus Conventional Radiotherapy in Head and Neck Cancer trial.[2] In addition, retrospective and prospective studies suggest improved locoregional control for skull-based tumors such as advanced nasopharynx and paranasal sinus cancer, whereby conventional techniques are unable to deliver tumoricidal doses while respecting dose limits to critical structures, including the optic pathways, retinas, frontal lobes, and brainstem, among others (**Figs. 1–3**).

In planning for RT, several contours are added to the planning CT scan, to specify the targets to be covered and the structures to be avoided. These contours are based on clinical and radiological findings, as well as knowledge of the likely patterns of spread, and taking into account uncertainties in patient setup and internal motion that may occur.[3]

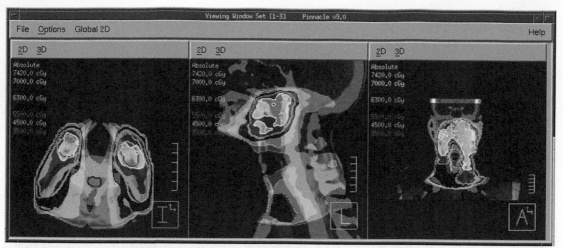

Fig. 1. Example of an IMRT plan for a patient with a locally advanced oropharyngeal cancer. Note how the surrounding normal structures, including the oral cavity, parotids, larynx, midbrain, and spine, are avoided, while treating the tumor and draining lymph nodes.

- Gross tumor volume (GTV)—The GTV is defined by the extent of visible tumor as defined by clinical evaluation and imaging of the tumor using CT, magnetic resonance imaging, or positron emission tomography. Multiple imaging modalities can be used to define the GTV, with the images "fused" with the planning CT scan in the treatment planning system.
- Clinical target volume (CTV)—The CTV extends beyond the GTV and accounts for potential microscopic spread of the tumor beyond the area defined by clinical examination and imaging.
- Internal target volume—The internal target volume accounts for the internal motion of tumors during treatment, for example, respiratory motion or motion with swallowing.
- Planning target volume (PTV)—The PTV extends beyond the CTV, to take into account the potential variations of treatment setup between fractions and/or organ motion during therapy. Daily patient positioning errors can occur during RT, ranging from 3 mm to 10 mm.[4,5] To compensate for this variation, a margin of 5 to 10 mm of normal tissue may be included in the PTV to ensure that the CTV is always within the PTV. However, this results in an increase in the dose of radiation administered to normal tissue in the PTV, which can significantly increase toxicity. Various techniques are being developed in an attempt to minimize the volume of normal tissue within the PTV, by reducing the setup error using image guidance.

- Organs at risk (OAR)—The OARs are normal tissues or organs in proximity to the PTV. These OARs are outlined so that the radiation dose can be constrained, to ensure that the delivered dose is less than the tolerance dose for that specific organ or tissue. If the OAR is a critical structure, such as the spinal cord or brainstem, an expansion may be added to the organ or tissue to ensure that the organ is protected from exposure to high doses of radiation.

To improve the accuracy and reproducibility of patient setup further, high-resolution on-board imaging is used to guide radiation delivery immediately before each radiation treatment. These images are compared with the images taken during the treatment planning process, and fine adjustments can be made to the patient's position. This process is termed image-guided radiation therapy. The imaging technologies used also include onboard orthovoltage radiograph imaging and cone-beam CT scanning.

RT planning generally uses a single-treatment plan based on the initial size and location of the tumor and the normal organs, as visualized on the simulation CT scan. The size and shape of the tumor, and of the surrounding normal tissues, can change significantly during the course of RT, usually due to shrinkage in response to RT and weight loss.[6] The relative locations of the tumor and normal organs may therefore change during treatment, resulting in a higher dose to normal tissue later in the course of the RT than is reflected in the initial plan.[7] This result can be mitigated by replanning part way through the course of treatment,

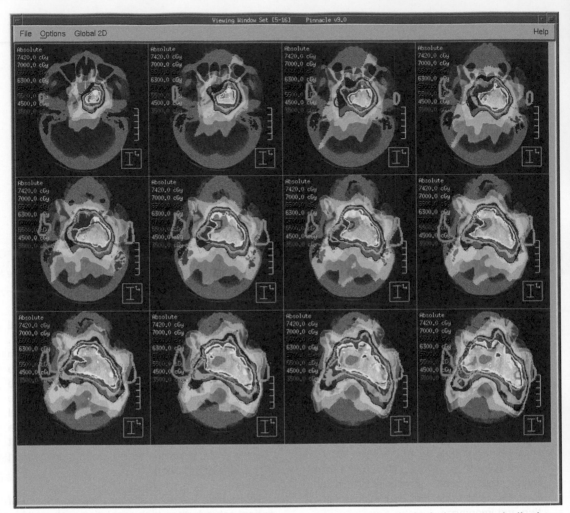

Fig. 2. Further CT slices with RT plan of the same patient demonstrating how the high-dose region (*yellow*) conforms the PTV (*outlined in red*), while minimizing the dose to the left and right parotid (*outlined in orange and green,* respectively) and other adjacent normal structures.

especially when a significant change in tumor size has occurred.[8] As a further refinement of image-guided radiation therapy, image-guided adaptive radiation therapy allows for adjustment of the radiation plan according to tumor size changes or normal organ shift during the course of the 6 to 7 weeks of treatment. By integrating image guidance data, such as cone beam CT, these changes can be detected during the treatment course, and thresholds can be established for the extent of changes that would justify replanning.[9] Due to concerns regarding possible interruptions in treatment during replanning, and the significant increase in workload and manpower required, this is not routinely done at this time.

When definitive RT is preceded by induction chemotherapy, appropriate imaging studies should be obtained before induction chemotherapy to serve as a reference for postinduction chemotherapy RT planning.[10] Changes in body weight, neck contours, and tumor volumes that occur during the induction chemotherapy may result in a smaller target volume if the postchemotherapy images only are used for treatment planning. With shrinkage of the tumor, however, there may still be viable tumor cells anywhere within the previously involved areas. The pretreatment primary tumor and gross nodal tumor volumes should therefore be used for treatment planning, and all structures involved by tumor before induction chemotherapy should be included in the final treatment plan, even if gross tumor is no longer identifiable.

Another technique for RT is brachytherapy, which involves an invasive procedure under general anesthetic, placing radioactive sources within or adjacent to the tumor. This procedure can be

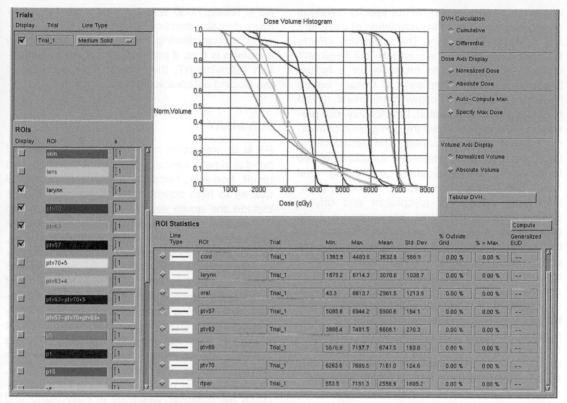

Fig. 3. Example of dose volume histogram used to evaluate the plan for the patient with a locally advanced oropharyngeal cancer, to ensure that the targets (tumor and draining lymph nodes) are treated to an adequate dose of radiation, while ensuring that the dose to the surrounding normal tissues does not exceed predetermined dose constraints.

achieved by using either an interstitial implant or an intracavitary device. Intracavitary brachytherapy involves placing the radiation source in the lumen of cavitary structures, such as the nasopharynx[11] or oral cavity. Brachytherapy can be used as a boost technique following external beam treatment or as the primary treatment in carefully selected small oral cavity or tonsillar tumors.[12,13] The advantage of brachytherapy is that it allows the delivery of high doses of radiation to the target and the sparing of surrounding tissues, due to the rapid exponential fall off of radiation dose around the source. Brachytherapy is, however, invasive and has the potential to cause severe late side effects, especially soft tissue necrosis and osteoradionecrosis. The risk of these complications is greatest in the areas immediately adjacent to the implant. Despite the documented increase in tumor control versus external beam RT alone, brachytherapy is not currently in widespread use for the treatment of head and neck cancer.

An emerging technology, stereotactic body radiotherapy mimics the effect of brachytherapy by using multiple converging external beam portals, creating steep dose falloffs into adjacent normal tissues. This highly conformal treatment is delivered in 3 to 8 high-dose fractions and requires a more rigorous immobilization than conventional treatment. This approach remains investigational for head and neck tumors, owing to potential late toxicities, including hemorrhage, soft tissue necrosis, and osteonecrosis. It has best been implemented for recurrent tumors in phase II single-institution protocols, alone or in combination with cytotoxic agents.[14]

TOXICITY FROM RT

Cancers of the head and neck arise from, or are in close proximity to, organs that are sensitive and important to quality of life. These tumors, as well as the side effects of treatment aimed at eradicating them, can interfere with the function of organs, such as the tongue or larynx, interfering with basic functions such as swallowing, taste, phonation. The toxicity from cancer therapy is categorized as acute or late based on the temporal relationship to treatment. Acute toxicity develops during or shortly after the completion of treatment and is usually temporary. The acute side effects typically start about 2 weeks into the treatment course and continue to progress for a further 2 weeks following completion of therapy before healing. By 3 weeks following treatment, acute toxicities are usually healed. Late toxicity may present months to years after the completion of treatment and is often permanent. The tissues of the head and neck have important functions related to breathing, communication, and eating. Oral intake can be compromised by mucositis, problems with swallowing (dysphagia and odynophagia), xerostomia, and alterations in taste (dysgeusia). Respiration and communication can be compromised by bulky tumors obstructing the airway, as well as from neuromuscular impairment secondary to tumors growth, or an edematous pharynx and/or larynx that can occur due to tumor or treatment. Patients may also experience skin toxicity from RT (and from epidermal growth factor receptor targeted agents such as cetuximab) neurotoxicity and ototoxicity from both commonly used chemotherapy agents (cisplatin) and radiation (brachial plexopathy), and dental complications from the effects of radiation dose to the mandible/maxilla and salivary glands. The most frequent long-term toxicities include xerostomia, due to damage to salivary glands. Fibrosis of tissues in the neck can result in induration and limitation in mobility. Damage to the muscles involved in mastication can result in trismus.

There are several methods that can be used to minimize the toxicity of RT. Measures such as avoiding direct sun exposure, hot water, tight collars, abrasion, and scratching of the skin can reduce the severity of skin toxicity. Radiation dermatitis is usually ameliorated by using emollients. Oropharyngeal mucositis typically causes pain and odynophagia, which can affect fluid and nutritional intake. Avoiding hot beverages and smoking cessation can reduce the severity of oropharyngeal mucositis. Saline mouth rinses, ice chips, and mouth rinses containing a local anesthetic, such as 2% viscous lidocaine, and systemic analgesics are used to provide short-term relief.

Dental health has a significant effect on post-treatment quality of life for patients with head and neck cancer.[15,16] The decrease in volume of saliva and changes in the quality of saliva induced by cancer treatment can alter the oral microbial flora, resulting in increased risk of subsequent dental caries. These patients frequently have poor pre-existing dentition, resulting in increased risks of complications from their cancer treatment.

As a result, head and neck patients frequently have dental extraction, often total dental clearance, before initiating treatment. One of the main concerns is that, if patients require dental extraction following RT, they are at increased risk of developing osteoradionecrosis.

SUMMARY

RT is an important modality in the treatment of head and neck cancers. Significant morbidity can result, however, because of exposure of normal tissues to high doses of RT. These side effects include the acute side effects occurring during and shortly after treatment, especially mucositis and dermatitis, and the risk of long-term toxicities, including dry mouth, fibrosis, dysphagia, and risk of osteonecrosis. Advances in RT planning and delivery, especially IMRT, can reduce the risk of these toxicities by ensuring that, whereas the tumor and draining lymph nodes are adequately treated, the surrounding organs and tissues at risk are avoided. Advances in technology including image guidance during treatment delivery can further improve the accuracy, and therefore, require a smaller margin around the tumor to account for potential variations in daily setup and positioning. All these advances help to improve the quality of life of cancer survivors.

REFERENCES

1. Lee N, Puri DR, Blanco AI, et al. Intensity-modulated radiation therapy in head and neck cancers: an update. Head Neck 2007;29(4):387.
2. Nutting CM, Morden JP, Harrington KJ, et al, PARSPORT Trial Management Group. Parotid-sparing intensity modulated versus conventional radiotherapy in head and neck cancer (PARSPORT): a phase 3 multicentre randomised controlled trial. Lancet Oncol 2011;12(2):127.
3. Prescribing, Recording and Reporting Photon Beam Therapy (Supplement to ICRU Report 50), ICRU Report 62. Bethesda, MD: ICRU; 1999.
4. Pisani L, Lockman D, Jaffray D, et al. Setup error in radiotherapy: on-line correction using electronic kilovoltage and megavoltage radiographs. Int J Radiat Oncol Biol Phys 2000;47(3):825.
5. Hong TS, Tomé WA, Chappell RJ, et al. The impact of daily setup variations on head-and-neck intensity-modulated radiation therapy. Int J Radiat Oncol Biol Phys 2005;61(3):779.
6. Piermattei A, Cilla S, D'Onofrio G, et al. Large discrepancies between planned and actually delivered dose in IMRT of head and neck cancer. A case report. Tumori 2007;93(3):319.

7. Vásquez Osorio EM, Hoogeman MS, Al-Mamgani A, et al. Local anatomic changes in parotid and submandibular glands during radiotherapy for oropharynx cancer and correlation with dose, studied in detail with nonrigid registration. Int J Radiat Oncol Biol Phys 2008;70(3):875.

8. Hansen EK, Bucci MK, Quivey JM, et al. Repeat CT imaging and replanning during the course of IMRT for head-and-neck cancer. Int J Radiat Oncol Biol Phys 2006;64(2):355.

9. Mageras GS, Mechalakos J. Planning in the IGRT context: closing the loop. Semin Radiat Oncol 2007;17(4):268.

10. Salama JK, Haddad RI, Kies MS, et al. Clinical practice guidance for radiotherapy planning after induction chemotherapy in locoregionally advanced head-and-neck cancer. Int J Radiat Oncol Biol Phys 2009;75(3):725.

11. Wang CC. Improved local control of nasopharyngeal carcinoma after intracavitary brachytherapy boost. Am J Clin Oncol 1991;14(1):5.

12. Mazeron JJ, Belkacemi Y, Simon JM, et al. Place of Iridium 192 implantation in definitive irradiation of faucial arch squamous cell carcinomas. Int J Radiat Oncol Biol Phys 1993;27(2):251.

13. Nag S, Cano ER, Demanes DJ, et al, American Brachytherapy Society. The American Brachytherapy Society recommendations for high-dose-rate brachytherapy for head-and-neck carcinoma. Int J Radiat Oncol Biol Phys 2001;50(5):1190.

14. Siddiqui F, Raben D, Lu JJ, et al. Emerging applications of stereotactic body radiation therapy for head and neck cancer. Expert Rev Anticancer Ther 2011; 11(9):1429–36.

15. Su YB, Vickers AJ, Zelefsky MJ, et al. Double-blind, placebo-controlled, randomized trial of granulocyte-colony stimulating factor during postoperative radiotherapy for squamous head and neck cancer. Cancer J 2006;12(3):182.

16. Staar S, Rudat V, Stuetzer H, et al. Intensified hyperfractionated accelerated radiotherapy limits the additional benefit of simultaneous chemotherapy–results of a multicentric randomized German trial in advanced head-and-neck cancer. Int J Radiat Oncol Biol Phys 2001;50(5): 1161.

The Role of Bisphosphonates in Medical Oncology and Their Association with Jaw Bone Necrosis

Ahmed Eid, MD[a],*, Jennifer Atlas, MD[b]

KEYWORDS

- Bisphosphonates • Bisphosphonate-related osteonecrosis of the jaw • Cancer • Jaw bone necrosis
- Multiple myeloma • Oncology

KEY POINTS

- Bisphosphonates can be used to treat patients with multiple myeloma or solid tumors with metastatic lesions to the bones.
- They can also be used to combat malignancy-associated metabolic disorders, such as hypercalcemia, and hormonal- and chemotherapy-induced osteoporosis.
- Bisphosphonate side effects include acute-phase Infusion reactions, kidney impairment, and bisphosphonate-related osteonecrosis of the jaw (BRONJ).
- The pathogenesis of BRONJ is multifactorial, involving remodeling suppression, osteoclast depression, angiogenesis disruption, and infection.
- The effect of oral pH may influence the propagation of BRONJ.
- Drugs that affect bone remodeling or angiogenesis may result in BRONJ-like symptoms.

Bisphosphonates, synthetic analogues to inorganic pyrophosphates found in the bone matrix, inhibit bone resorption. Bisphosphonates and their related effects on the jaw have been established since 2001.

THE ROLE OF BISPHOSPHONATES IN MEDICAL ONCOLOGY

Bisphosphonates are used in many clinical situations to treat conditions causing bone resorption, such as metastatic bone disease (particularly seen with multiple myeloma, breast cancer, and prostate cancer), osteoporosis, hypercalcemia, and Paget disease.

Mechanism of Action

Bisphosphonates, synthetic analogues to inorganic pyrophosphates found in the bone matrix, work by inhibiting bone resorption.[1] They do not repair existing bone damage, but help prevent formation of new lytic lesions. They do so through several mechanisms of action, including attaching to hydroxyapatite-binding sites on bony surfaces to impair osteoclast activity, decreasing the development of osteoclast progenitor cells, and promoting apoptosis of osteoclasts.[2–4]

Normal bone growth and maintenance involve a tightly coupled process of bone resorption by osteoclasts and deposition by osteoblasts.

Disclosures: No conflict of interest to disclose.
[a] General Oncology, The University of Texas MD Anderson Cancer Center, 1515 Holcombe Boulevard, Unit 0462, Houston, TX 77030, USA; [b] Hematology and Oncology, Comprehensive Cancer Center of Wake Forest School of Medicine, Medical Center Boulevard, Winston-Salem, NC 27157, USA
* Corresponding author.
E-mail address: aeid@mdanderson.org

Oral Maxillofacial Surg Clin N Am 26 (2014) 231–237
http://dx.doi.org/10.1016/j.coms.2014.01.009
1042-3699/14/$ – see front matter © 2014 Elsevier Inc. All rights reserved.

Bisphosphonates inhibit the resorption of bone by accumulating in resorption lacunae located near osteoclasts. At the time of bone resorption, bisphosphonates are released locally and absorbed by osteoclasts; this inhibits osteoclasts maturation and leads to apoptosis.[3]

Types of Bisphosphonates

There are three different groups of bisphosphonates: those without nitrogen substitution (eg, etidronate, clodronate), aminobisphosphonates (eg, pamidronate, alendronate), and bisphosphonates substituted at nitrogen (eg, ibandronate, risedronate, zoledronate). The bisphosphonates substituted at nitrogen are the more potent inhibitors of bone resorption and act by inhibiting farnesyl pyrophosphate synthase, which causes cytoskeletal abnormalities in the osteoclast and an accumulation of bisphosphonates substituted at nitrogen farnesyl pyrophosphate precursor, isopentenyl pyrophosphate. Isopentenyl pyrophosphate binds to a receptor that allows the release of tumor necrosis factor-α, which may be responsible for the acute-phase reaction seen with bisphosphonates.[5–8] The non–nitrogen-containing bisphosphonates act by causing apoptosis of osteoclasts when metabolites from the bisphosphonates are exchanged with the terminal pyrophosphate moiety of ATP, which prevents the ATP from being used as an energy source.[7]

Administration and Side Effects

Route of administration

Bisphosphonates can be administered either orally or intravenously. Because bisphosphonates have poor oral absorption (approximately 1%), they are absorbed best on an empty stomach. Two advantages of intravenous bisphosphonate administration are that it has a short infusion time and greater bioavailability than oral bisphosphonates, and that intravenous bisphosphonates are often given monthly, which increases patient compliance. Not all bisphosphonates have the same potency. Intravenous bisphosphonates, which are used in patients with multiple myeloma, are more potent than oral bisphosphonates, which are used in patients with osteoporosis.

Side effects

The side effects that can be seen with intravenous or oral bisphosphonate use include acute-phase infusion reactions, kidney impairment, and osteonecrosis of the jaw.[9] During therapy with bisphosphonates, patients should maintain good oral hygiene, have regular dental examinations, and avoid dental procedures. Side effects can be seen with either oral or intravenous bisphosphonate use, but are more common with intravenous administration because of the greater potency of the drugs. Bisphosphonates do not repair existing bone damage, but help prevent formation of new lytic lesions. Oral bisphosphonates can cause gastrointestinal side effects, such as gastritis and diarrhea.[10]

Absorption and half-life

Regardless of route of administration, approximately 70% of the absorbed bisphosphonate is cleared by the kidneys, and the other 30% is absorbed by the bone.[2] The exact half-lives of bisphosphonates are unknown, but they are thought to remain in the bone for years.[11]

Bisphosphonates in Multiple Myeloma

Based on several prospective, randomized controlled trials and two systematic reviews, bisphosphonates are used to treat patients with multiple myeloma to reduce pain and the risk of skeletal-related events.[12–16] Approximately 60% of patients with multiple myeloma have lytic lesions at the time of diagnosis.

Bisphosphonate treatment is generally well tolerated, but patients require periodic monitoring for complications, such as renal insufficiency, nephrotic syndrome, electrolyte abnormalities, and osteonecrosis of the jaw.[17] Laboratory tests that should be followed include serum creatinine, calcium, and magnesium levels. Patients undergoing treatment with bisphosphonates for multiple myeloma should have a 24-hour urine assessment every 3 to 6 months to screen for albuminuria.[17] If the albuminuria is greater than 500 mg in 24 hours, the bisphosphonate should be temporarily stopped.[17,18] This side effect occurs more frequently with pamidronate because it causes glomerular damage; in contrast, zoledronic acid damages the renal tubules.[19–21]

Steroids are routinely used as part of the treatment regimen in multiple myeloma and as an antiemetic given with chemotherapy, which also increases the risk of osteonecrosis of the jaw, as described later, and steroid-induced osteoporotic bone density loss. Before initiating therapy, patients should be evaluated for comorbidities that would require bisphosphonate dosing adjustments.

There are limited data concerning the optimal duration of treatment with bisphosphonates for multiple myeloma. In the absence of evidence from randomized clinical trials, the suggested dosing of bisphosphonates is monthly for a 2-year period; consideration is then given to stopping bisphosphonates in those with responsive or stable disease.[12,17,22–24] Therapy should be reinitiated if new skeletal-related events occur after cessation of the bisphosphonate.

Bisphosphonates in Solid Tumors

Bisphosphonates are also used to treat patients with solid tumors. Many solid tumors can metastasize to the bone, with the most common being breast and prostate cancer. Bone metastases cause many complications that significantly increase the morbidity in patients with these advanced cancers, including pathologic bone fractures; the need for surgery or radiation therapy for symptomatic relief; electrolyte disturbances, such as hypercalcemia; cancer treatment-related bone loss; nerve compression; and neurologic dysfunction.[18,25–27]

In breast cancer, chemotherapy can induce premature ovarian failure, which is a risk factor for decreased bone density; in prostate cancer, androgen-deprivation therapy is a risk factor for decreased bone density.[25] A review of patients with metastatic breast cancer before the routine use of bisphosphonates revealed that more than 50% developed skeletal-related events during their disease course.[28] Additional data suggest that in patients with breast cancer not treated with a medication to inhibit osteoclast activity, on average, a skeletal-related event is observed every 3 to 4 months in patients with lytic bone lesions.[29]

Bisphosphonates should be started in patients with cancer only after bone metastasis is distinguished on imaging. Bone metastases are best detected with imaging, such as radiographs, bone scans, and magnetic resonance imaging. Radiographs reveal lucencies or dark spots in the bone but often do not identify bone metastases until the cancer is advanced. However, bone scans and computed tomography scans are sensitive for detecting early metastases and magnetic resonance. However, magnetic resonance imaging is best for recognizing neurologic compromise.[27,30]

Bisphosphonates are used as part of the treatment regimen for other solid tumor malignancies, such as lung, kidney, stomach, bladder, uterus, thyroid, colon, and rectal cancers. The clinical trial data available for solid tumors, such as lung cancer, are more limited than the data available for breast and prostate cancer. Bisphosphonates have been demonstrated to improve quality of life by reducing bone pain associated with lytic lesions.[31,32] In a placebo-controlled trial, 773 patients with skeletal metastases from solid tumors other than breast and prostate (including non–small cell and small cell lung, renal cell, thyroid, and head and neck cancers) were assigned to receive either zoledronic acid or a placebo.[15,31,33]

Patients receiving bisphosphonates had not only a reduced incidence of skeletal-related events but also a longer time to first lytic lesion.

Bisphosphonates in Metabolic Disorders

Other important uses for bisphosphonates include the treatment of osteoporosis and hypercalcemia. Less potent oral bisphosphonates with reduced doses are used to treat osteoporosis in postmenopausal women and steroid-induced osteoporosis to decrease osteoporotic fractures (40%–70% reduction in fractures compared with placebo) while reducing the chance of bisphosphonate-related side effects. Risk factors for osteoporosis in noncancer patients include smoking, excessive alcohol intake, low calcium, vitamin D deficiency, genetic history, decreased weight-bearing exercise, and medication side effects (proton pump inhibitors, anticoagulants, certain anticonvulsants).[25] An added risk associated with malignancy is hypercalcemia. Elevated calcium and alkaline phosphatase levels can be detected through blood work and suggest lytic bone lesions in a patient with cancer.[17,27]

Other Bone-Modifying Agents

Denosumab is another bone-modifying agent with the ability to inhibit osteoclasts. Denosumab is a highly specific human IgG_2 monoclonal antibody that specifically binds receptor activator of nuclear factor kappa B, blocking the binding of receptor activator of nuclear factor kappa B ligand. Denosumab targets the receptor activator of nuclear factor kappa B ligand to block the formation of osteoclasts.[34] Side effects include hypocalcemia, hypophosphatemia, fatigue, and nausea, and as with bisphosphonates, there is a risk of osteonecrosis of the jaw. Several studies have demonstrated that patients receiving denosumab have a longer period free of skeletal-related events than do patients receiving bisphosphonates.[30,35,36] Patients receiving bisphosphonates or denosumab should take calcium and vitamin D supplementation as long as there are no contraindications, such as significant renal impairment or failure. An important distinction between bisphosphonates and denosumab is that denosumab is not cleared by the kidneys, so dose adjustments and renal monitoring are not required.

In summary, bisphosphonates can be used to treat patients with multiple myeloma or solid tumors with metastatic lesions to the bones, and to combat malignancy-associated metabolic disorders, such as hypercalcemia and hormonal and chemotherapy-induced osteoporosis. There are many ongoing studies further investigating the potency, optimal dosing regimens, and side effects of bisphosphonates to determine the effective duration of use and when to initiate treatment with bisphosphonates.

ASSOCIATED RISK OF JAW BONE NECROSIS WITH BISPHOSPHONATES

Bisphosphonates and their related effects on the jaws have been established since 2001.[37] There are multiple hypotheses for the pathogenesis of bisphosphonate-related osteonecrosis of the jaw (BRONJ); however, the exact mechanism by which jaw necrosis forms is still not completely understood. BRONJ is diagnosed when a patient currently or previously treated with a bisphosphonate has exposed bone in the maxillofacial region, with no history of radiation therapy to the jaws.[38]

Pathogenesis

The pathogenesis of BRONJ is multifactorial, involving remodeling suppression, osteoclast depression, angiogenesis dysruption, and infection. The suppression of osteoclasts causes a decrease in bone remodeling of the jaws. The jaws' normal physiologic remodeling is rapid (10–20 times faster than the cortex of the iliac crest) and as a result, the negative effects of bisphosphonates are seen in the jaws earlier than in other bones.

A decrease in angiogenesis is a known contributor to the pathogenesis of osteonecrosis and radio-osteonecrosis. Therefore, it would make sense that bisphosphonate use would contribute to BRONJ; bisphosphonates have been shown to decrease angiogenesis and are being explored as tumor growth suppressors. When remodeling and vasculature suppression are combined with dentoalveolar surgery, the chance of BRONJ is drastically increased. After tooth extraction, the extraction site undergoes a series of healing steps, which include initial clot formation, conversion of clot to granulation tissue, and formation of connective tissue and osteoid. The site is then filled with woven bone and remodeled into lamellar bone.[39] Consequently, if osteoclasts are suppressed, the remodeling of woven bone does not proceed normally, and combined with defective angiogenesis, all aspects of healing are delayed, which ultimately may lead to BRONJ. Furthermore, it has been shown that patients taking the medication bevacizumab, a recombinant human monoclonal antibody that binds to vascular endothelial growth factor and inhibits angiogenesis, develop BRONJ-like symptoms.[40]

Local tissue pH has recently been shown to have relevance to the pathogenesis of BRONJ.

Bisphosphonates substituted at nitrogen bind to bone at a neutral pH and are released in an acidic environment. This pharmacologic mechanism is observed in the resorption lacunas during bone resorption, where acidic pH increases the dissociation between bisphosphonates and hydroxyapatite. In the presence of infection or trauma in the jaw, the pH in local tissue decreases, which can then lead to an increase in release of bisphosphonate, leading to BRONJ. This hypothesis is further supported by the fact that bisphosphonates without nitrogen substitution, which are not affected by a more acidic pH, do not normally contribute to BRONJ.[41]

Bisphosphonates are not the only treatment of diseases with high bone turnover or metastasis; new inhibitors of osteoclast differentiation and function are available.[42,43] Because of the similar mechanism of action of denosumab, patients have been shown to develop BRONJ-like symptoms.[44]

Many patients taking bisphosphonates have other comorbidities and may be on glucocorticoids. Although glucocorticoids are beneficial for certain pathologic processes, they have negative effects on the skeleton by decreasing the production of osteoclasts and osteoblasts, increasing apoptosis of osteoblasts, and increasing the lifespan of osteoclasts.[45,46] Alone, glucocorticoids are the most common cause of nontraumatic osteonecrosis, developing in 9% to 40% of patients on long-term glucocorticoid therapy.[47] Glucocorticoids and bisphosphonates taken concomitantly have been shown to exacerbate the effects on bone remodeling and to result in BRONJ that appears faster, is more severe, and is more unpredictable to treat.[48] **Fig. 1** illustrates a severe case of BRONJ in a patient receiving glucocorticoids and bisphosphonate demonstrating the seriousness of this disease's consequences and the complicated treatment involved.

Aside from their mechanism of action, bisphosphonates remain in the body for extended periods of time. This leads to the further complication of how to manage and prevent BRONJ when treating a patient who has received bisphosphonates in the past. Drug holidays are suggested as a means of prevention of BRONJ, but it is unclear how long bisphosphonates remain in the body, and a patient cannot wait when an acute invasive procedure is needed.

In summary, the pathogenesis of BRONJ is multifactorial and still under investigation. Currently, drugs with mechanisms of action involving remodeling suppression, osteoclast depression, and decreasing angiogenesis are under investigation for causing BRONJ-like symptoms. Further studies are needed to determine the effective length of use

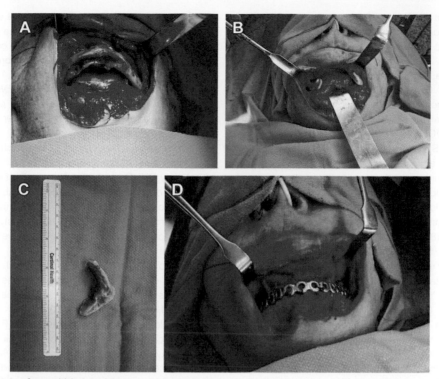

Fig. 1. Necrosis of mandible in a 65-year-old woman with 15-year history of oral bisphosphonate and steroid use. She presented with a submental cutaneous fistula and a nonhealing extraction site 1 year after dental extraction. (*A*) Necrosis extends through the inferior border of the mandible. (*B*) Necrotic area of the mandible excised, debridement of bone continued until vital bone reached. (*C*) Excised specimen. (*D*) Defect reconstructed with a reconstruction plate. (*Courtesy of* Dr. Nagi Damian, Oral & Maxillofacial Surgery, University of Texas Health Science Center at Houston, Houston, TX.)

of biphosponates and the efficacy of drug holidays to prevent BRONJ.

ACKNOWLEDGMENTS

The authors thank Timothy C. Woernley III DS4, University of Texas School of Dentistry, and Amelia Scholtz, PhD and Melissa Burkett, Department of Scientific Publications, The University of Texas MD Anderson Cancer Center.

REFERENCES

1. Rogers MJ, Gordon S, Benford HL, et al. Cellular and molecular mechanisms of action of bisphosphonates. Cancer 2000;88(Suppl 12):2961–78.
2. Fleisch H. Bisphosphonates: mechanisms of action. Endocr Rev 1998;19(1):80–100.
3. Hughes DE, Wright KR, Uy HL, et al. Bisphosphonates promote apoptosis in murine osteoclasts in vitro and in vivo. J Bone Miner Res 1995;10(10):1478–87.
4. Rodan GA, Fleisch HA. Bisphosphonates: mechanisms of action. J Clin Invest 1996;97(12):2692–6.
5. Dunford JE. Molecular targets of the nitrogen containing bisphosphonates: the molecular pharmacology of prenyl synthase inhibition. Curr Pharm Des 2010; 16(27):2961–9.
6. Rogers MJ. From molds and macrophages to mevalonate: a decade of progress in understanding the molecular mode of action of bisphosphonates. Calcif Tissue Int 2004;75(6):451–61.
7. Russell RG, Watts NB, Ebetino FH, et al. Mechanisms of action of bisphosphonates: similarities and differences and their potential influence on clinical efficacy. Osteoporos Int 2008;19(6):733–59.
8. Terpos E, Sezer O, Croucher PI, et al. The use of bisphosphonates in multiple myeloma: recommendations of an expert panel on behalf of the European Myeloma Network. Ann Oncol 2009;20(8): 1303–17.
9. Diel IJ, Bergner R, Grötz KA. Adverse effects of bisphosphonates: current issues. J Support Oncol 2007;5(10):475–82.
10. Major PP, Lipton A, Berenson J, et al. Oral bisphosphonates: a review of clinical use in patients with bone metastases. Cancer 2000;88(1):6–14.
11. Kimmel DB. Mechanism of action, pharmacokinetic and pharmacodynamic profile, and clinical applications of nitrogen-containing bisphosphonates. J Dent Res 2007;86(11):1022–33.

12. Berenson JR, Rosen LS, Howell A, et al. Zoledronic acid reduces skeletal-related events in patients with osteolytic metastases. Cancer 2001;91(7):1191–200.

13. Kyle RA. The role of bisphosphonates in multiple myeloma. Ann Intern Med 2000;132(9):734–6.

14. Mhaskar R, Redzepovic J, Wheatley K, et al. Bisphosphonates in multiple myeloma: a network meta-analysis. Cochrane Database Syst Rev 2012;(5):CD003188.

15. Rosen LS, Gordon D, Kaminski M, et al. Long-term efficacy and safety of zoledronic acid compared with pamidronate disodium in the treatment of skeletal complications in patients with advanced multiple myeloma or breast carcinoma: a randomized, double-blind, multicenter, comparative trial. Cancer 2003;98(8):1735–44.

16. Ross JR, Saunders Y, Edmonds PM, et al. Systematic review of role of bisphosphonates on skeletal morbidity in metastatic cancer. BMJ 2003;327(7413):469.

17. Kyle RA, Yee GC, Somerfield MR, et al. American Society of Clinical Oncology 2007 clinical practice guideline update on the role of bisphosphonates in multiple myeloma. J Clin Oncol 2007;25(17):2464–72.

18. Dunstan CR, Felsenberg D, Seibel MJ. Therapy insight: the risks and benefits of bisphosphonates for the treatment of tumor-induced bone disease. Nat Clin Pract Oncol 2007;4(1):42–55.

19. Berenson JR, Yellin O, Crowley J, et al. Prognostic factors and jaw and renal complications among multiple myeloma patients treated with zoledronic acid. Am J Hematol 2011;86(1):25–30.

20. Markowitz GS, Fine PL, Stack JI, et al. Toxic acute tubular necrosis following treatment with zoledronate (Zometa). Kidney Int 2003;64(1):281–9.

21. Perazella MA, Markowitz GS. Bisphosphonate nephrotoxicity. Kidney Int 2008;74(11):1385–93.

22. Durie BG. Use of bisphosphonates in multiple myeloma: IMWG response to Mayo Clinic consensus statement. Mayo Clin Proc 2007;82(4):516–7 [author reply: 517–8].

23. Lacy MQ, Dispenzieri A, Gertz MA, et al. Mayo Clinic consensus statement for the use of bisphosphonates in multiple myeloma. Mayo Clin Proc 2006; 81(8):1047–53.

24. Rosen LS, Gordon D, Kaminski M, et al. Zoledronic acid versus pamidronate in the treatment of skeletal metastases in patients with breast cancer or osteolytic lesions of multiple myeloma: a phase III, double-blind, comparative trial. Cancer J 2001; 7(5):377–87.

25. Gralow JR, Biermann JS, Farooki A, et al. NCCN Task Force Report: bone health in cancer care. J Natl Compr Canc Netw 2009;7(Suppl 3):S1–32 [quiz: S33–5].

26. Mehrotra B, Ruggiero S. Bisphosphonate complications including osteonecrosis of the jaw. Hematology Am Soc Hematol Educ Program 2006;356–60.

27. Van Poznak CH, Temin S, Yee GC, et al. American Society of Clinical Oncology executive summary of the clinical practice guideline update on the role of bone-modifying agents in metastatic breast cancer. J Clin Oncol 2011;29(9):1221–7.

28. Domchek SM, Younger J, Finkelstein DM, et al. Predictors of skeletal complications in patients with metastatic breast carcinoma. Cancer 2000;89(2): 363–8.

29. Coleman RE. Uses and abuses of bisphosphonates. Ann Oncol 2000;11(Suppl 3):179–84.

30. Henry DH, Costa L, Goldwasser F, et al. Randomized, double-blind study of denosumab versus zoledronic acid in the treatment of bone metastases in patients with advanced cancer (excluding breast and prostate cancer) or multiple myeloma. J Clin Oncol 2011;29(9):1125–32.

31. Aapro M, Abrahamsson PA, Body JJ, et al. Guidance on the use of bisphosphonates in solid tumours: recommendations of an international expert panel. Ann Oncol 2008;19(3):420–32.

32. Wardley A, Davidson N, Barrett-Lee P, et al. Zoledronic acid significantly improves pain scores and quality of life in breast cancer patients with bone metastases: a randomised, crossover study of community vs hospital bisphosphonate administration. Br J Cancer 2005;92(10):1869–76.

33. Rosen LS, Gordon D, Tchekmedyian NS, et al. Long-term efficacy and safety of zoledronic acid in the treatment of skeletal metastases in patients with nonsmall cell lung carcinoma and other solid tumors: a randomized, phase III, double-blind, placebo-controlled trial. Cancer 2004;100(12): 2613–21.

34. West H. Denosumab for prevention of skeletal-related events in patients with bone metastases from solid tumors: incremental benefit, debatable value. J Clin Oncol 2011;29(9):1095–8.

35. Fizazi K, Carducci M, Smith M, et al. Denosumab versus zoledronic acid for treatment of bone metastases in men with castration-resistant prostate cancer: a randomised, double-blind study. Lancet 2011;377(9768):813–22.

36. Stopeck AT, Lipton A, Body JJ, et al. Denosumab compared with zoledronic acid for the treatment of bone metastases in patients with advanced breast cancer: a randomized, double-blind study. J Clin Oncol 2010;28(35):5132–9.

37. Ruggiero SL. Bisphosphonate-related osteonecrosis of the jaw (BRONJ): initial discovery and subsequent development. J Oral Maxillofac Surg 2009; 67(Suppl 5):13–8.

38. Ruggiero SL, Dodson TB, Assael LA, et al. American Association of Oral and Maxillofacial Surgeons position paper on bisphosphonate-related osteonecrosis of the jaws–2009 update. J Oral Maxillofac Surg 2009;67(Suppl 5):2–12.

39. Allen MR, Burr DB. The pathogenesis of bisphosphonate-related osteonecrosis of the jaw: so many hypotheses, so few data. J Oral Maxillofac Surg 2009;67(Suppl 5):61–70.

40. Estilo CL, Fornier M, Farooki A, et al. Osteonecrosis of the jaw related to bevacizumab. J Clin Oncol 2008;26(24):4037–8.

41. Otto S, Hafner S, Mast G, et al. Bisphosphonate-related osteonecrosis of the jaw: is pH the missing part in the pathogenesis puzzle? J Oral Maxillofac Surg 2010;68(5):1158–61.

42. Geusens P. Emerging treatments for postmenopausal osteoporosis: focus on denosumab. Clin Interv Aging 2009;4:241–50.

43. Reddy GK, Mughal TI, Roodman GD. Novel approaches in the management of myeloma-related skeletal complications. Support Cancer Ther 2006; 4(1):15–8.

44. Aghaloo TL, Felsenfeld AL, Tetradis S. Osteonecrosis of the jaw in a patient on Denosumab. J Oral Maxillofac Surg 2010;68(5):959–63.

45. Weinstein RS, Jilka RL, Parfitt AM, et al. Inhibition of osteoblastogenesis and promotion of apoptosis of osteoblasts and osteocytes by glucocorticoids. Potential mechanisms of their deleterious effects on bone. J Clin Invest 1998;102(2):274–82.

46. O'Brien CA, Jia D, Plotkin LI, et al. Glucocorticoids act directly on osteoblasts and osteocytes to induce their apoptosis and reduce bone formation and strength. Endocrinology 2004;145(4):1835–41.

47. Weinstein RS. Glucocorticoid-induced osteonecrosis. Endocrine 2012;41(2):183–90.

48. Chiu CT, Chiang WF, Chuang CY, et al. Resolution of oral bisphosphonate and steroid-related osteonecrosis of the jaw–a serial case analysis. J Oral Maxillofac Surg 2010;68(5):1055–63.

Nuclear Medicine Imaging Studies in the Diagnosis of Head and Neck Disease

Steve Chiang, MD

KEYWORDS

- PET/CT • Drug-induced osteonecrosis of the jaw (DIONJ) • Nuclear medicine imaging • FDG

KEY POINTS

- Positron emission tomography/computed tomography has proven utility in oncology imaging.
- Fluorodeoxyglucose positron emission tomography/computed tomography may be useful for delineating drug-induced osteonecrosis of the jaw.

INTRODUCTION TO PET/CT IMAGING

The detection and localization of positron decay within the body are the means by which positron emission tomography (PET) images are created. Positron decay is a form of radioactive decay, which is the process by which unstable atoms spontaneously convert to a more stable form with a lower overall energy. The resultant energy emission releases radioactive energy that is used to create medically useful images. Most positron-emitting isotopes are produced in a cyclotron.

Previously, cyclotrons were located only in major research institutions and academic centers, because of the high cost and resources needed to operate and maintain a cyclotron. However, in recent years, cyclotrons have been purchased by commercial companies to produce medically useful isotopes, specifically, positron-emitting isotopes. Also, current cyclotron size has become significantly more convenient than past versions (**Fig. 1**). In particular, the radiotracer fluorodeoxyglucose (FDG) has led the way in PET imaging in routine clinical oncology.[1] PET/computed tomography (CT) scanners combine PET imaging with an in-line CT scanner for accurate localization of PET tracer uptake and comprise most of the current PET scanner sales.

As with all images generated in nuclear medicine, PET attempts to map a biologic process related to the tracer injected. Often the image represents functional metabolic activity, most often for oncologic indications.[1,2] Current radiotracers used for PET/CT imaging are numerous, but only one is used in routine clinical practice at this time, 18F-FDG. This tracer is simply a glucose molecule with one oxygen atom substituted with radioactive fluorine-18 (18F), which is a positron-emitting radioisotope produced in a cyclotron. Metabolic functional imaging with the radiotracer FDG attempts to map the glucose utilization pattern of the bodily tissues. FDG (and nonradioactive glucose) enters cells actively, depending on cell surface transporters (GLUT-1 and -2). Often, these are up-regulated in malignant and inflammatory cells, leading to greater uptake within the cell, and subsequently, leading to abnormalities on PET imaging. Malignant cells also "metabolically trap" FDG, because these cells are unable to metabolize FDG, whereas inflammatory cells are "hypermetabolic" and subsequently use more glucose. Other substrates may be incorporated into radiotracers, for example, fatty acids, amino acids, and charged particles.[3] The development of new radiotracers is an exciting part of nuclear medicine, which will drive future application

Radiology, The Methodist Hospital, 6565 Fannin Street, Houston, TX 77030, USA
E-mail address: sbchiang@tmhs.org

Oral Maxillofacial Surg Clin N Am 26 (2014) 239–245
http://dx.doi.org/10.1016/j.coms.2014.02.001
1042-3699/14/$ – see front matter © 2014 Elsevier Inc. All rights reserved.

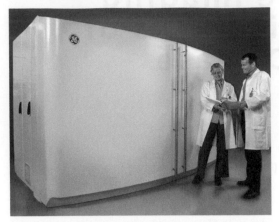

Fig. 1. Typical relative dimensions of a clinical cyclotron. (*Courtesy of* General Electric Company; with permission.)

of PET imaging and image-guided therapy. Advances in radiochemistry have made tracer development an exciting topic, which will become more apparent in the near future.

After intravenous injection, FDG distributes throughout the body, creating a physiologic pattern. Glucose is a substrate for nearly every cell in the human body, especially the brain, heart, liver, and skeletal muscle. These organs provide most of the background activity on PET scans. Normal tissue, including bone marrow, undergoing physiologic metabolism accounts for the remaining background activity on PET scans. FDG has been shown to accumulate avidly in inflammatory cells[4] as well as neoplastic cells. The mechanism of uptake in both inflammatory and neoplastic cells has been well studied.[5] Once activated, inflammatory cells demonstrate markedly increased metabolism, leading to increased glucose utilization and subsequent increased activity on a PET scan. In theory, normal osseous FDG uptake could be used as a biomarker for viable mandible in preparation for surgical resection of diseased bone. However, abnormal osseous uptake on an FDG-PET scan almost always signifies pathologic abnormality, such as metastatic disease, infection, or other inflammation, particularly, drug-induced

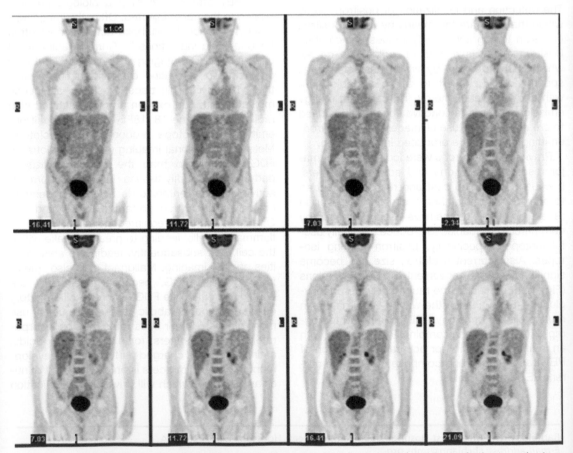

Fig. 2. Normal, physiologic whole-body FDG distribution. Note high background activity in the brain and urinary bladder. (*Courtesy of* General Electric Company; with permission.)

osteonecrosis of the jaw (DIONJ). Other bone-specific agents could also be used. In particular, 18F sodium fluoride also shows promise, because it allows for PET.[6] Single-photon emitters, such as Tc-99m methylenediphosphonate, have been described in the use of localization of DIONJ,[6,7] but in the authors' opinion, uptake is too nonspecific and image resolution is not sufficient to be of use clinically.

TECHNICAL ASPECTS OF PET IMAGING

During the tracer uptake period after injection, the patient should remain as calm as possible. Physiologic uptake will always be present in the skeletal muscle, including the muscles of mastication. To keep this at a minimum, muscle activity should be kept minimal. Current policy is to place the patient in a quiet room on a stretcher to avoid activity. Trips to the rest room are allowed, as is water to drink. Obviously, carbohydrate meals are to be avoided during the uptake period. Another potential pitfall is talking or chewing during the uptake period, especially in patients being evaluated for DIONJ or head and neck pathologic abnormality. Uptake by the oropharynx can be quite intense normally, and when combined with increased uptake within the retropharyngeal and glossal muscles, often leads to suboptimal scans of this area. For surgical planning purposes, obviously, false positive uptake is undesirable. Fortunately, with the advent of PET/CT scanners,

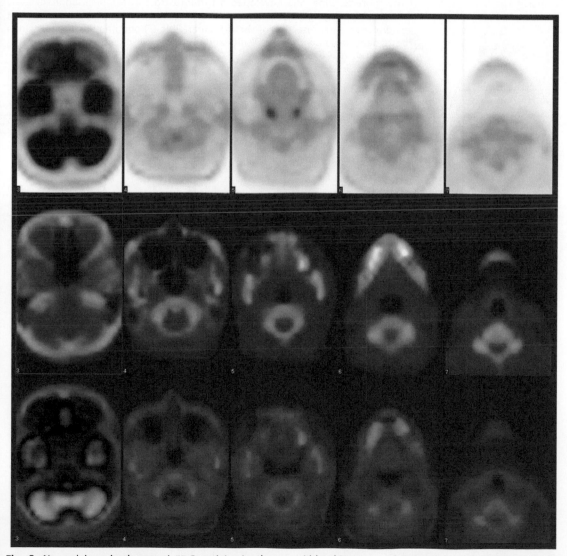

Fig. 3. Normal low, background FDG activity in the mandible. (*Courtesy of* General Electric Company; with permission.)

the rate of false positive uptake has decreased because of the ability to localize uptake accurately to benign lymphoid tissue rather than pathologic abnormality.[8]

Technical issues related to scanning are relatively simple. Paramount to imaging the head and neck is minimization of motion artifact (ie, movement between the PET and CT portions of the study), which leads to so-called misregistration artifacts and could potentially lead to errors in interpretation. Metallic artifacts are also a problem with PET/CT scanning in which the CT scan is use for attenuation mapping.[9,10] Metal leads to artificially increased attenuation coefficients for a given area, leading to overcorrection during the attenuation correction process and has been known to

cause false positive uptake on a scan.[11] Fortunately, with PET/CT fusion, these artifacts are easily identified on the corresponding CT images. Intravenous contrast also poses the same issues, due to the high measured metallic density in an anatomic area, which would not otherwise be metallic in density. These artifacts are also easy to identify on combined PET/CT scans.

TYPICAL IMAGES

Physiologic distribution of FDG can be described as simply glucose metabolism in the body. Expected areas of glucose metabolism include the brain, heart, and visceral organs, such as the liver and spleen. As described above, skeletal muscle

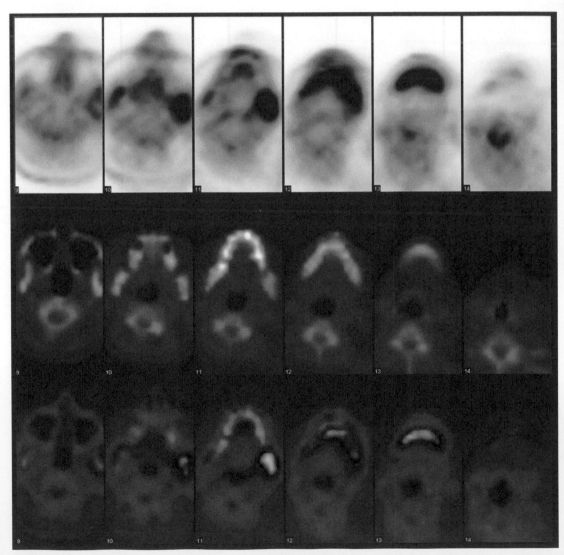

Fig. 4. Appearance of DIONJ. Note areas of diffuse and focal FDG uptake correlating with apparent sclerosis on the CT. (*Courtesy of* General Electric Company; with permission.)

activity should be at a minimum if patient preparation has been adequate. **Fig. 2** shows the typical distribution of FDG on a whole-body scan. Note the normal, minimal background activity in the osseous structures. Unless there is underlying pathologic abnormality or a bone marrow stimulating pharmaceutical (eg, granulocyte colony-stimulating factor or granulocyte-macrophage colony-stimulating factor) has been administered, background bone marrow activity is minimal. As of the writing of this article, the most commonly approved oncologic indications for whole-body PET/CT scanning under Medicare guidelines are as follows: solitary pulmonary nodule, staging/restaging nonsmall cell lung cancer, thyroid cancer, head and neck cancer staging/restaging, colorectal cancer staging/restaging, esophageal cancer staging/restaging, breast cancer staging/restaging, melanoma staging/restaging, and lymphoma staging/restaging.[2] Unfortunately, PET is not typically approved for the evaluation of the mandible unless performed for one of the above-mentioned diagnoses.

PET IMAGING IN DIONJ

FDG PET/CT imaging has potential in separating areas of active DIONJ from unaffected normal mandibular marrow. **Fig. 3** shows the normal appearance of the mandible on PET/CT imaging. As described previously,[6] the authors' experience has shown that areas of active DIONJ will show increased uptake relative to normal marrow (**Fig. 4**). Note the marked changes seen on CT

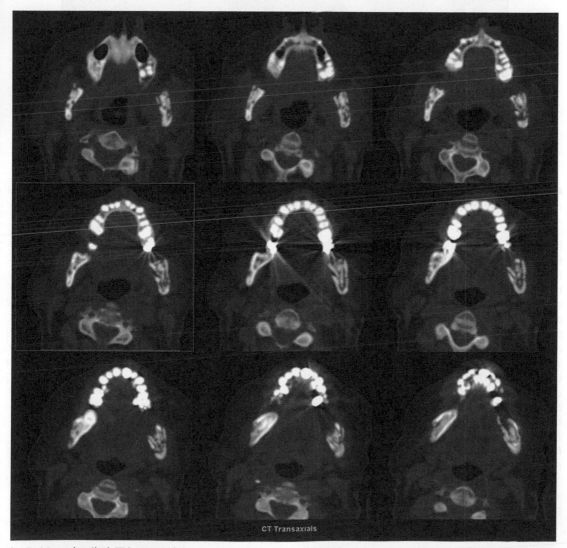

CT Transaxials

Fig. 5. More detailed CT images of the previous patient show a bony sequestrum in the left mandible, commonly seen in DIONJ. (*Courtesy of* General Electric Company; with permission.)

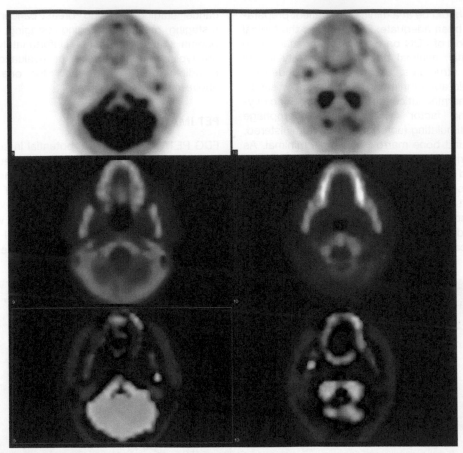

Fig. 6. Appearance of osteomyelitis. Note multiple foci of FDG uptake. Radiographically, this can appear identical to DIONJ. (*Courtesy of* General Electric Company; with permission.)

(**Fig. 5**). Abnormal uptake likely reflects active inflammatory cells within the bony matrix. FDG PET imaging has the potential to guide surgery by delineating healthy mandible from affected mandible. Potential pitfalls would include the inability to discriminate between DIONJ and metastatic disease as well as the possibility of concomitant osteomyelitis of the mandible, both of which will show abnormally increased FDG uptake in the mandible (**Fig. 6**). In these settings, accurate clinical history and examination are paramount, because there is often a history of other bone metastases. Additional imaging, such as magnetic resonance imaging and CT, may also be useful. Future tracer development may also play a larger role in imaging DIONJ.

REFERENCES

1. Rohren EM, Turkington TG, Coleman RE. Clinical applications of PET in oncology. Radiology 2004;231: 305–32.

2. Juweid ME, Cheson BD. Positron emission tomography and assessment of cancer therapy. N Engl J Med 2006;354:496–507.

3. Shiue CY, Welch MJ. Update of PET radiopharmaceuticals: life beyond fluorodeoxyglucose. Radiol Clin North Am 2004;42:1033–53.

4. Deichen JT, Prante O, Gack M, et al. Uptake of [18F] fluorodeoxyglucose in human monocyte-macrophages in vitro. Eur J Nucl Med Mol Imaging 2003;30:267–73.

5. Pauwels EK, Ribeiro MJ, Stoot JH, et al. FDG accumulation and tumor biology. Nucl Med Biol 1998;25: 317–22.

6. Wilde F, Steinhoff K, Frerich B, et al. Positron-emission tomography imaging in the diagnosis of bisphosphonate-related osteonecrosis of the jaw. Oral Surg Oral Med Oral Pathol Oral Radiol Endod 2009;107(3):412–9.

7. Morag Y, Morag-Hezroni M, Jamadar D, et al. Bisphosphonate-related osteonecrosis of the jaw: a pictorial review. Radiographics 2009;29:1971–84.

8. Sureshbabu W, Mawlawi O. PET/CT imaging artifacts. J Nucl Med Technol 2005;33:156–61.

9. Heiba SI, Luo J, Sadek S, et al. Attenuation-correction induced artifact in F-18 FDG PET imaging following total knee replacement. Clin Positron Imaging 2000;3:237–9.

10. Bujenovic S, Mannting F, Chakrabarti R, et al. Artifactual 2-deoxy-2-[(18)F]fluoro-D-glucose localization surrounding metallic objects in a PET/CT scanner using CT-based attenuation correction. Mol Imaging Biol 2003;5:20–2.

11. Goerres GW, Schmid DT, Eyrich GK. Do hardware artifacts influence the performance of head and neck PET scans in patients with oral cavity squamous cell cancer? Dentomaxillofac Radiol 2003;32:365–71.

Pharmacologic Modalities in the Treatment of Osteoradionecrosis of the Jaw

James Anthony McCaul, PhD, FRCS(OMFS), FRCS, FDSRCPS[a,b,*]

KEYWORDS

- Osteoradionecrosis • Radiation-induced fibroatrophy • Pentoxifylline • Tocopherol • Clodronate

KEY POINTS

- Managing osteoradionecrosis (ORN) of the facial bones is a challenge in maxillofacial head and neck surgical practice.
- Changes in understanding of ORN of the jaws has led to new studies using novel therapeutic modalities to manage this disorder.
- These treatment regimens may allow medical management to replace major reconstructive surgery for some patients who have already undergone chemoradiotherapy or combined modality therapy for head and neck cancer.

INTRODUCTION

Osteoradionecrosis (ORN) of the jaws was first described in the 1920s and remains the most problematic complication occurring after the use of radiotherapy to treat head and neck cancer.[1] The condition has been defined as exposed and necrotic bone associated with ulcerated or necrotic soft tissue that persists for greater than 3 months in an area that has been previously irradiated, and is not caused by tumor recurrence.[2] According to the current medical literature, approximately 20.0% (range, 0.9%–35.0%) of patients have radiotherapy as part of their head and neck cancer treatment.[3] This incidence may be declining.[4] The condition affects the mandible most frequently, and diagnosis depends on clinical features, including a history of exposure to greater than 50 Gy of ionizing radiation. Symptoms include pain, trismus, and dysesthesia. Clinical signs include ulceration and/or necrosis of the oral mucosa, exposure of underlying bone, malodor, and, in advanced stages, ulceration of overlying skin and pathologic fracture.[5]

PATHOGENESIS

Four hypotheses have been described for the development of ORN. Watson and Scarborough[6] first described the sequence of radiation exposure, local injury, and infection as a possible cause, and this hypothesis was further popularized by Meyer.[7]

Later Marx[8] described the "Three-H" hypothesis: wherein the area shows a hypocellular, hypoxic, and hypovascular state. This condition is thought to be consequent to microvasculature damage, resulting in endarteritis, thrombosis, and vessel obliteration.

A more recently described hypothesis is that of suppression of osteoclast mediated bone turnover, wherein irradiation-induced loss of osteoclast function results in the clinical features described earlier. This idea is supported by the evidence from antiresorptive therapy–related osteonecrosis of the jaws, which occurs after administration of bisphosphonates and other antiresorptive agents in some patients.

Delanian and Lefaix[9,10] proposed a fourth hypothesis of fibroatrophic bone change in 2004

[a] Maxillofacial/Head and Neck Surgery, The Royal Marsden Hospital, London, UK; [b] UK RCS/BAOMS/Saving Faces Maxillofacial Surgical Specialty Lead for Research, London, UK
* Maxillofacial/Head and Neck Surgery, The Royal Marsden Hospital, London, UK.
E-mail address: jim.mccaul@mac.com

Oral Maxillofacial Surg Clin N Am 26 (2014) 247–252
http://dx.doi.org/10.1016/j.coms.2014.02.002

based on enhanced understanding of the cellular and molecular biology of the histopathologic features seen in ORN. Earlier, in 1998, the first report emerged of bone healing in a patient with ORN of the sternum after receiving radiotherapy for carcinoma of the breast 29 years previously treated with pharmacologic therapy based upon this new hypothesis. With this hypothesis, bone and soft tissue damage is proposed to be caused by radiation-induced fibrosis, and this has been summarized by Lyons and Ghazali.[11] Three phases of tissue injury are described, which mirror those in healing of chronic traumatic wounds[12]: the initial predominantly acute inflammatory phase with endothelial changes, a second phase of abnormal fibroblast activity with extracellular matrix disruption, and a third late fibroatrophic phase. At this late phase, the healed tissues are friable and undergo late reactivation of the acute inflammatory response after injury.

In the proposed fibroatrophic mechanism, the key event in ORN progression is described as activation and dysregulation of fibroblast activity, resulting in tissue atrophy and fibrosis. Radiation-induced endothelial injury initiates

cytokine release, including tumor necrosis factor α (TNF-α); fibroblast growth factor β; platelet-derived growth factor; interleukin (IL) 1, 2, and 4; connective tissue growth factor; and transforming growth factor β1 (TGF-β1). This process produces a predominance of the myofibroblast phenotype, with attendant high rates of cellular proliferation and release of abnormal extracellular matrix (ECM) components.[13] These myofibroblasts also demonstrate impaired ability to breakdown the abnormal ECM. This is shown diagrammatically in **Fig. 1**. This fibroblast process is similarly described in fibrotic processes in the lungs and liver after tissue injury of various types.[14]

Ionizing radiation produces osteoblast cell death and prevents repopulation of this cellular component of bone. Together with excess myofibroblast proliferation and abnormal ECM formation, a reduction in bony hard tissue matrix and an excess of fibrous tissue is described. Four possible mechanisms of bony destruction are suggested by Delanian and colleagues[15] in an article describing microradiographic analysis of ORN bone. These mechanisms are progressive macrophage-mediated osteoclast loss with no accompanying

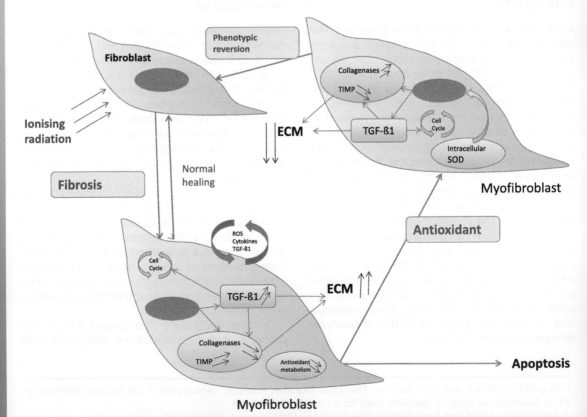

Fig. 1. Activation and dysregulation of fibroblast activity. (*Modified from* Delanian S, Lefaix JL. The radiation-induced fibroatrophic process: therapeutic perspective via the antioxidant pathway. Radiother Oncol 2004;73(2):119–31.)

osteogenesis; periosteocytic lysis; extensive de-mineralization; and accelerated bone aging.

Therefore, after radiotherapy, bone has reduced numbers of viable cells, is poorly vascularized, and is fibrosed compared with normal healthy bone. Apoptosis of the myofibroblast component reduces cellularity further.[14] This tissue is then at risk of the development of ORN after any physical or chemical trauma, which induces the late acute inflammatory response described earlier. **Fig. 2** summarizes this process.

PHARMACOLOGIC AGENTS IN ORN MANAGEMENT

The initial infection-based hypothesis resulted in treatment based on antibiotic therapy and surgical

debridement. Later work by Marx described bacteria as a superinfection rather than as being involved in pathogenesis, but nonetheless antibiotic therapy in acute episodes of pyogenic infection in ORN, guided by microbiologic samples and culture and sensitivity assays, remains a cornerstone of treatment.

Hyperbaric Oxygen Therapy

Hyperbaric oxygen therapy is still widely used for ORN prevention and management, although this practice has had recent challenges.[5,16,17] In the United Kingdom, the Medicines and Healthcare Products Regulatory Agency considers hyperbaric oxygen a medicinal product, and therefore inspect trials involving this modality (eg, the HOPON

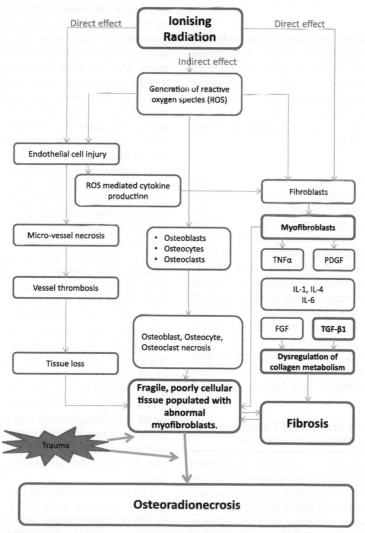

Fig. 2. The ionizing radiation–induced fibroatrophic process. (*Modified from* Lyons A, Ghazali N. Osteoradionecrosis of the jaws: current understanding of its pathophysiology and treatment. Br J Oral Maxillofac Surg 2008;46(8):653–60.)

trial; Professor Richard Shaw, personal communication). This modality is discussed elsewhere in this issue.

Pentoxifylline and Tocopherol

Pentoxifylline

Pentoxifylline is a methylxanthine derivative that has multiple effects considered advantageous in ORN management, including vascular dilatation and increased erythrocyte flexibility effects, both of which enhance blood flow. Furthermore, pentoxifylline has anti–TNF-α activity and is thought to reduce the cytokine cascade driving the ORN process. It has also been shown to reduce proliferation of dermal fibroblasts and limit ECM production by these cells. In vitro experiments have also shown promotion of collagenase activity in these cells.[18]

Tocopherol

Tocopherol is a fat-soluble vitamin (vitamin E) and is a weak antioxidant agent. Therefore, tocopherol is capable of scavenging reactive oxygen species involved in the pathogenesis of ORN, wherein they induce cell membrane peroxidation among other deleterious effects. Tocopherol also shows partial inhibition of TGF-β1 and an antifibrotic effect mediated by procollagen genes.[11]

Clodronate

This agent is a first-generation, nonnitrogenous bisphosphonate approved for use in osteoporosis, hyperparathyroidism, hypercalcemia of malignancy, and multiple myeloma. Clodronate reduces bone resorption through reducing osteoclast numbers and activity. It is also known to reduce inflammatory cytokines IL-1β, IL-6, and TNF-α. Although bisphosphonates are clearly implicated in antiresorptive therapy–related osteonecrosis of the jaws, clodronate has been used in French studies of severe ORN cases and been described as effective (see next section).[18,19] Notably and uniquely among this group of agents, clodronate also has been shown to act on osteoblasts to increase bone formation[20] and reduce fibroblast proliferation.[21]

Pentoxifylline and Tocopherol Combined Therapy With or Without Clodronate

Experiments in vitro and animal studies have been unable to show that either pentoxifylline or tocopherol alone can reduce reactive oxygen species. Combination therapy with these agents has been described in several radiation-associated tissue injury studies, including small placebo-controlled randomized trials.[22,23] These reports show benefit for combination therapy over placebo treatment

and single-agent therapy, and also that rebound tissue injury can occur if treatment is too short (<3 months).

Delanian and colleagues[18,19] have described 2 phase II trials of combined therapy for ORN of the mandible. In the first, 18 consecutive patients were treated with pentoxifylline and tocopherol. Each had at least 13.4 mm of exposed mandibular bone and all had been prescribed pentoxifylline, 400 mg twice daily and tocopherol, 1000 IU orally for 6 to 24 months.[18] The worst affected cases (n = 8) were also given clodronate, 1600 mg daily for 5 days per week. The second trial,[19] published in 2011, reported on 54 patients who received radiation for head and neck cancer a mean of 5 years before the onset of ORN. In this report, the term PENTOCLO was coined for the treatment regimen including all 3 agents. This treatment regimen had evolved to combined pentoxifylline and tocopherol as described earlier, with clodronate, 1600 mg given 5 days per week, and prednisone, 20 mg with ciprofloxacin given on the other 2 days. This study showed that prolonged treatment (16 ± 9 months) was safe and well tolerated. All patients in the study experienced improvement, with an exponential progressive and significant reduction in exposed bone ($P<.0001$). A total of 36 patients underwent spontaneous sequestrectomy during the course of treatment. All patients in this series were shown to experience complete recovery in a median time of 9 months. The investigators concluded that the treatment is safe and effective, and recommended that a randomized controlled trial be conducted.

In a retrospective series of 12 patients treated with pentoxifylline and tocopherol without clodronate, McLeod and colleagues[1] show more modest treatment outcomes. These patients were treated for a mean of 14.8 months (range, 4.0–46.0 months). One patient stopped treatment because of side effects to pentoxifylline, and 3 reported difficulty in swallowing the large pentoxifylline tablets, and resorted to crushing them, against pharmaceutical advice. Epstein scoring showed that 5 patients improved, 5 were unchanged, and 2 had become worse. Three patients deteriorated and subsequently underwent resection and composite free flap reconstruction surgery. These authors acknowledge that they did not use clodronate for any of the cases in this short retrospective series.

The Bradford Teaching Hospitals series reports on 18 patients with ORN after radiotherapy or chemoradiotherapy administered as part of head and neck cancer therapy (McCaul and colleagues, unpublished data, 2014). These prospectively followed patients all received

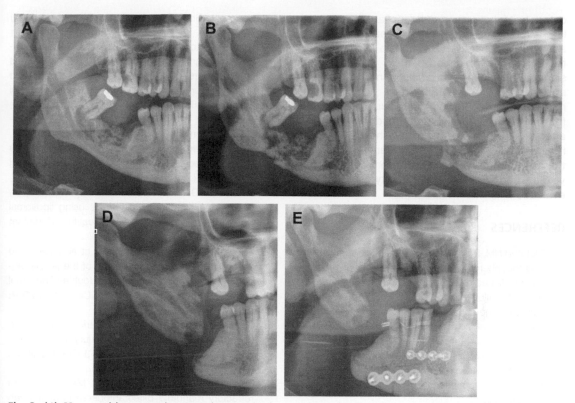

Fig. 3. (*A*) 62-year-old man underwent chemoradiotherapy for a T4,N3 right oropharynx squamous carcinoma. This tumor exhibited complete response and was followed up according to protocol. (*B*) In November of 2010 he presented complaining of pain from the right lower third of his face and had exposed bone and pus discharging intraorally. No evidence was seen of new primary cancer at this site and the bone exposure persisted for more than 3 months. He was managed initially with antibiotic therapy and local intraoral measures. He then commenced pentoxifylline, 400 mg twice daily and tocopherol, 1000 IU daily. His ORN remained quiescent but progressed. (*C*) Autosequestrectomy occurred after this time and his symptoms settled to a firm fibrous nonunion with good function. He did not require surgical intervention. (*D*) The patient later developed a new primary cancer of the right lateral tongue, which required lip split mandibulotomy for access to resect and reconstruct, and this healed without incident. (*E*) He remained on pentoxifylline and tocopherol throughout this process.

combined therapy with pentoxifylline and tocopherol only, and not clodronate for similar reasons as in the cases reported by McLeod and colleagues.[1] Two patients could not tolerate therapy and did not continue with the agents, and 16 continued with therapy. ORN resolved in 7 patients (44% of patients completing therapy); in 3 with medical therapy alone and in 3 with medical therapy and surgical debridement. Three patients received hyperbaric oxygen therapy as part of ORN management. In 1 patient, medical therapy resulted in a symptom-free fibrous bony union of the right body of the mandible (**Fig. 3**). No adverse events have been associated with vitamin E and pentoxifylline therapy in the Bradford series. None of these patients have experienced progression on therapy, and none have required major resection and reconstruction for ORN in the past 8 years. The Bradford center treats 240 new head and neck cancers per year,

two-thirds of which require radiotherapy or chemoradiotherapy as part of treatment for cure.

SUMMARY

Recent changes in understanding of the pathogenesis of ORN have led to the emergence of some exciting new pharmacologic therapies. Uptake of these agents has been generally slow worldwide, despite the success of the Delanian group[18,19] in France, perhaps partly because of the previous acceptance that ORN of the mandible is a surgical disease for which hyperbaric oxygen therapy can be of utility. However, there is a clear reluctance among surgeons who are faced with an increasing burden of antiresorptive agent–induced osteonecrosis of the jaw to introduce clodronate into the therapeutic armamentarium for ORN. Clodronate seems to be unique among the bisphosphonate group in that it can stimulate osteoblast function and reduce inflammatory cytokine expression. Small, randomized studies have shown the effectiveness of the pentoxifylline tocopherol combination versus placebo and single-agent therapy in radiation-induced trauma at other body sites. It is clear, however, that high-quality, randomized, controlled trial evidence for this approach is currently lacking for ORN affecting the human mandible. The PENTOCLO regimen offers an exciting, potentially curative therapy for mandibular ORN for some cancer survivors, and requires high-quality clinical trial evaluation.

REFERENCES

1. McLeod NM, Pratt CA, Mellor TK, et al. Pentoxifylline and tocopherol in the management of patients with osteoradionecrosis, the Portsmouth experience. Br J Oral Maxillofac Surg 2012;50(1):41–4.

2. Harris M. The conservative management of osteoradionecrosis of the mandible with ultrasound therapy. Br J Oral Maxillofac Surg 1992;30(5):313–8.

3. Cheriex KC, Nijhuis TH, Mureau MA. Osteoradionecrosis of the jaws: a review of conservative and surgical treatment options. J Reconstr Microsurg 2013; 29(2):69–75.

4. Clayman L. Clinical controversies in oral and maxillofacial surgery: part two. Management of dental extractions in irradiated jaws: a protocol without hyperbaric oxygen therapy. J Oral Maxillofac Surg 1997;55(3):275–81.

5. Shaw RJ, Dhanda J. Hyperbaric oxygen in the management of late radiation injury to the head and neck. Part I: treatment. Br J Oral Maxillofac Surg 2011;49(1):2–8.

6. Watson WL, Scarborough JE. Osteoradionecrosis in intraoral cancer. Am J Roentgenol 1938;40:524–38.

7. Meyer I. Infectious diseases of the jaws. J Oral Surg 1970;28(1):17–26.

8. Marx RE. Osteoradionecrosis: a new concept of its pathophysiology. J Oral Maxillofac Surg 1983; 41(5):283–8.

9. Delanian S, Lefaix JL. The radiation-induced fibroatrophic process: therapeutic perspective via the antioxidant pathway. Radiother Oncol 2004;73(2):119–31.

10. Delanian S, Lefaix JL. Complete healing of severe osteoradionecrosis with treatment combining pentoxifylline, tocopherol and clodronate. Br J Radiol 2002;75(893):467–9.

11. Lyons A, Ghazali N. Osteoradionecrosis of the jaws: current understanding of its pathophysiology and treatment. Br J Oral Maxillofac Surg 2008;46(8): 653–60.

12. Vozenin-Brotons MC, Milliat F, Sabourin JC, et al. Fibrogenic signals in patients with radiation enteritis are associated with increased connective tissue growth factor expression. Int J Radiat Oncol Biol Phys 2003;56(2):561–72.

13. Dambrain R. The pathogenesis of osteoradionecrosis. Rev Stomatol Chir Maxillofac 1993;94(3):140–7.

14. Riley PA. Free radicals in biology: oxidative stress and the effects of ionizing radiation. Int J Radiat Biol 1994;65(1):27–33.

15. Delanian S, Baillet F, Huart J, et al. Successful treatment of radiation-induced fibrosis using liposomal Cu/Zn superoxide dismutase: clinical trial. Radiother Oncol 1994;32(1):12–20.

16. Annane D, Depondt J, Aubert P, et al. Hyperbaric oxygen therapy for radionecrosis of the jaw: a randomized, placebo-controlled, double-blind trial from the ORN96 study group. J Clin Oncol 2004; 22(24):4893–900.

17. Shaw RJ, Butterworth C. Hyperbaric oxygen in the management of late radiation injury to the head and neck. Part II: prevention. Br J Oral Maxillofac Surg 2011;49(1):9–13.

18. Delanian S, Depondt J, Lefaix JL. Major healing of refractory mandible osteoradionecrosis after treatment combining pentoxifylline and tocopherol: a phase II trial. Head Neck 2005;27(2):114–23.

19. Delanian S, Chatel C, Porcher R, et al. Complete restoration of refractory mandibular osteoradionecrosis by prolonged treatment with a pentoxifylline-tocopherol-clodronate combination (PENTOCLO): a phase II trial. Int J Radiat Oncol Biol Phys 2011; 80(3):832–9.

20. Fromigue O, Body JJ. Bisphosphonates influence the proliferation and the maturation of normal human osteoblasts. J Endocrinol Invest 2002;25(6):539–46.

21. Fast DK, Felix R, Dowse C, et al. The effects of diphosphonates on the growth and glycolysis of connective-tissue cells in culture. Biochem J 1978; 172(1):97–107.

22. Delanian S, Porcher R, Rudant J, et al. Kinetics of response to long-term treatment combining pentoxifylline and tocopherol in patients with superficial radiation-induced fibrosis. J Clin Oncol 2005;23(34): 8570–9.

23. Delanian S, Porcher R, Balla-Mekias S, et al. Randomized, placebo-controlled trial of combined pentoxifylline and tocopherol for regression of superficial radiation-induced fibrosis. J Clin Oncol 2003;21(13):2545–50.

Magnetic Resonance Imaging (MRI) in the Diagnosis of Head and Neck Disease

Emilio P. Supsupin Jr, MD[a],*, Nagi M. Demian, MD, DDS[b,c]

KEYWORDS

- Perineural spread • Brachial plexus • Orbital cellulitis • Head and neck disease • MRI

KEY POINTS

- Magnetic resonance imaging (MRI) is the modality of choice to identify intracranial extension and perineural spread from a head and neck primary tumor.
- Perineural spread is a form of metastatic disease in which primary tumors spread along neural pathways.
- Orbital cellulitis is a sight-threatening, and potentially life-threatening condition. Urgent imaging is performed to assess the anatomic extent of disease, including postseptal, cavernous sinus, and intracranial involvement, and to identify orbital abscesses that require exploration and drainage.
- MRI is useful the evaluation of the brachial plexus.

INTRODUCTION

Magnetic resonance imaging (MRI) is a proven and useful tool for the diagnosis, evaluation, and follow-up of diseases of the head and neck.[1] It is a multiplanar imaging method based on an interaction between radiofrequency electromagnetic fields and certain nuclei in the body (usually hydrogen nuclei) after placement of the body in a strong magnetic field. MRI differentiates between normal and abnormal tissues, providing a sensitive examination to detect disease. This sensitivity is based on the high degree of inherent contrast due to variations in the magnetic relaxation properties of different tissues, both normal and diseased, and the dependence of the MRI signal on these tissue properties.[2,3]

The benefits, advantages/disadvantages, and contraindications to MRI are summarized in **Box 1** and **Table 1**.[1,2] All patients should be screened for possible contraindications to MRI before scanning.[1,2]

APPROACH

A case-based approach highlighting the crucial role of MRI in the diagnosis of head and neck conditions is presented. More importantly, the impact of MRI on clinical decision-making and management is emphasized. The major applications of MRI in the head and neck, encompassing masses, congenital anomalies, vascular lesions, skull base imaging, and brachial plexus evaluation are represented by these cases.

[a] Department of Diagnostic and Interventional Imaging, University of Texas Health Science Center at Houston, 6431 Fannin Street, Houston, TX 77030, USA; [b] Oral & Maxillofacial Surgery Department, The University of Texas School of Dentistry, Lyndon B. Johnson Hospital, UT Annex 112 B, 5656 Kelly, Houston, TX 77026, USA; [c] The Externship Program, Dental Branch at UTHSC, UT Annex 112 B, 5656 Kelly, Houston, TX 77026, USA
* Corresponding author.
E-mail address: Emilio.P.Supsupin@uth.tmc.edu

Oral Maxillofacial Surg Clin N Am 26 (2014) 253–269
http://dx.doi.org/10.1016/j.coms.2014.03.002

APPLICATIONS

Neoplasms and Masses

MRI is the modality of choice to identify intracranial or perineural spread from a head or neck primary tumor.[1] MRI is superior in staging nasopharyngeal

Table 1
General benefits/advantages and disadvantages of MRI include but not limited to the following[1,2]

Advantages	Disadvantages
Three-dimensional depiction of a lesion	Clinical scenarios that may require sedation
Assessment of bone marrow	Contraindications to magnetic field exposure
Detection of subtle soft tissue contrast	Artifacts from metallic objects in the head and neck
Assessment of deep tissue planes	Long scan times (compared with CT)
No ionizing radiation (compared with CT)—particularly beneficial in pediatric patients	Risk of (NSF) nephrogenic systemic fibrosis (rare)
Ability to image patients with iodine contrast allergy	
Improved soft tissue resolution	

carcinoma because of its ability to detect tumor invasion of the skull base and intracranial extension (**Fig. 1**).[4,5]

MRI plays a crucial role in the diagnosis of perineural spread. Perineural spread is a form of metastatic disease in which primary tumors spread along neural pathways.[6] Nerves act as conduits that transmit tumor from a primary site to a deeper structure. Head and neck cancers can leave the primary tumor mass and travel antegradely and retrogradely along nerves to reemerge at deeper intracranial destinations.[7,8] The distinction between perineural invasion and perineural spread is important. Perineural invasion is a pathologic term describing microscopic perineural or endoneural tumor that is impossible to diagnose radiologically. Perineural invasion is confined to the main tumor mass. In contradistinction, perineural spread is separate from the main bulk of the tumor and is detectable on imaging. Cranial nerves V and VII are most commonly involved because of their extensive distribution.[8,9] Once tumors reach the cavernous sinus, additional cranial nerves may be involved.[8,9] Recognition of this mode of spread is crucial because of its adverse therapeutic and prognotic implications. Many treatment failures are attributed to unrecognized perineural tumor spread. Overall, perineural spread negatively impacts prognosis and jeopardizes long-term survival.

MRI findings of perineural tumor spread include thickening and enhancement of the nerve after gadolinium administration, widening of the neural foramen, and loss of fat surrounding the nerve. Enhancement of the nerve must be interpreted with caution in the absence of thickening or foraminal changes, because occasionally, the presence of extensive perineural vascular plexus may promote avid contrast uptake (seen as intense enhancement on MRI).[6,9–11] **Figs. 2–4** illustrate perineural spread involving multiple cranial nerves.

MRI is excellent in the characterization of soft tissues and may potentially provide histologic insight. For example, pleomorphic adenoma is typically hyperintense (bright) on T2-weighted MRI sequences, with sharp demarcation from the adjacent normal parotid tissue (**Fig. 5**).[12–16] MRI is useful in the characterization of acquired lesions such as ranulas. Ranulas are typically well-defined, homogeneously hypointense (dark) on T1-weighted MRI sequences and high signal on T2-weighted images (**Fig. 6**).[17]

Infections

In general, MRI is preferred for orbital imaging because of the absence of ionizing

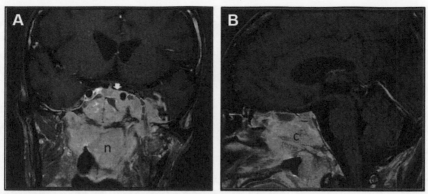

Fig. 1. Nasopharyngeal carcinoma with skull base invasion and intracranial extension: (*A*) Coronal postcontrast MRI: tumor invades the cavernous sinus and encases the left internal carotid artery (*red arc* and *red arrow*). Tumor extends into the lateral aspect of the sella (*yellow arrow*). There is infiltration and breach of the dura with enhancement of the base of the temporal lobe, indicating parenchymal invasion (*blue arc*). There is extensive tumor in the nasopharynx (n) with contiguous spread in the adjacent soft tissues in the masticator spaces bilaterally. (*B*) Sagittal postcontrast MRI: diffuse infiltration of the marrow cavity of the clivus (c). With skull base infiltration and intracranial extension, this case is clearly nonsurgical. This illustrates the impact of MRI in clinical decision-making and management approach to NPCA (nasopharyngeal carcinoma).

radiation.[18–20] MRI is helpful in the detection of intracranial complications of orbital infection. Orbital cellulitis is a sight-threatening, and potentially life-threatening condition. Urgent imaging is indicated to assess the anatomic extent of disease, including postseptal, cavernous sinus, and intracranial involvement, and to identify orbital abscesses that require exploration and

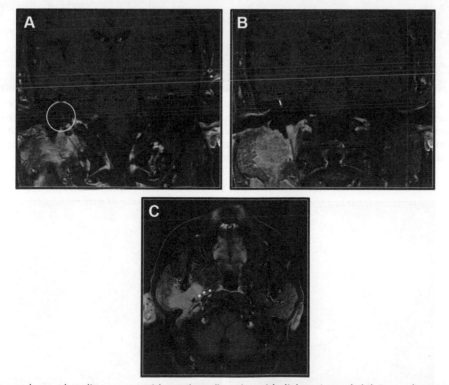

Fig. 2. Perineural spread: malignant parotid neoplasm (lymphoepithelial carcinoma): (*A*) Coronal postcontrast MRI, thickening and enhancement of the mastoid segment of the facial nerve (*circle*). (*B*) Coronal postcontrast MRI, tumor replacing a large portion of the parotid gland Geniculate ganglion (*arrow*). (*C*) Axial postcontrast MRI showing perineural spread with linear enhancement along the expected course of the auriculotemporal nerve (*yellow arrows*).

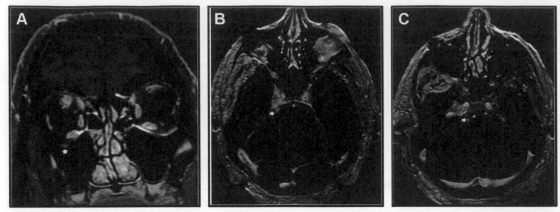

Fig. 3. Perineural spread: orbital squamous cell carcinoma (*red arrow* on *A*) with intracranial extension through perineural spread into V2 and cisternal segments/root entry zones of CN V and VI. (*A*) Coronal postcontrast MRI, thickened and enhancing infraorbital nerve (*yellow arrow*). (*B*) Axial postcontrast MRI, thickening and enhancement of the cisternal segment/root entry zone (*arrow*) of CN V. (*C*) Axial postcontrast MRI, thickening and enhancement of the cisternal segment/root entry zone (*arrow*) of CN VI.

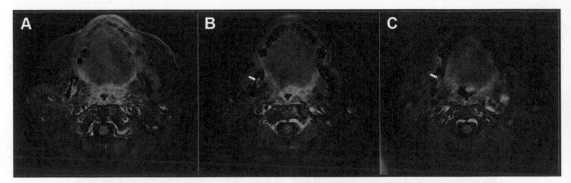

Fig. 4. Perineural spread in breast cancer: A 62-year-old Hispanic woman with known breast cancer, presented with chin numbness. (*A*) Axial postcontrast MRI demonstrating nodular enhancement at the entrance of the right inferior alveolar nerve with widening of the mandibular foramen (*red arrow*). (*B, C*) Contiguous slices show enhancement along the course of the right inferior alveolar nerve (*yellow arrows*). (*Courtesy of* Scott Benjamin Serlin, MD, University of Texas Health Science Center, Houston, TX.)

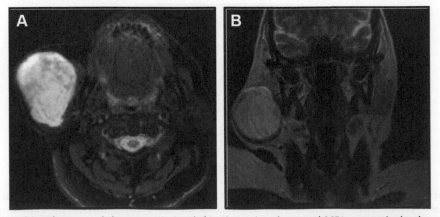

Fig. 5. Pleomorphic adenoma of the parotid gland: (*A, B*) Axial and coronal MRI, respectively, show a markedly hyperintense mass replacing almost the entirety of the right parotid gland with a thin rim of residual tissue peripherally. Marked T2 hyperintensity is a classic MRI feature of pleomorphic adenoma.

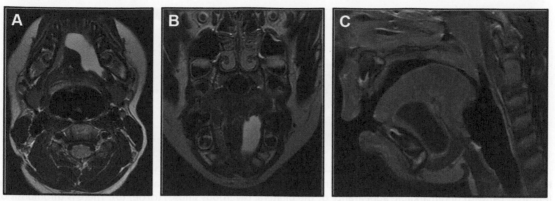

Fig. 6. Simple ranula: (*A, B*) Axial and coronal T2-weighted sequences, respectively, show a lobulated hyperintense lesion confined to the sublingual space. (*C*) Sagittal T1 postcontrast image demonstrates lack of intrinsic enhancement.

drainage.[1,21–23] MRI provides excellent contrast resolution in the orbit and is a powerful imaging technique to answer these questions.[21–23] Multiplanar capability and high spatial resolution allow MRI to provide details on the extent of disease, including involvement of important anatomic structures such as vessels (**Fig. 7**). Diffusion-weighted MRI is recently advocated for patients unable to receive contrast because of renal issues (**Fig. 8**).

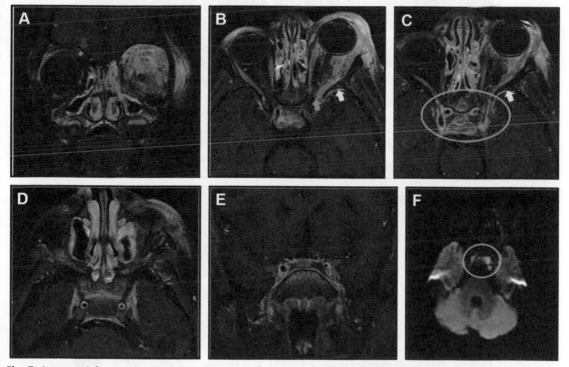

Fig. 7. Intracranial extension and complications of orbital infection: (*A*) Infection/inflammatory changes in the left orbit. Note the indistinct left superior ophthalmic vein, suggesting thrombosis. The right superior ophthalmic vein is normal (*red arrow*). (*B*) Extension of postseptal infection/inflammatory process into the orbital apex (*green arrow*) with focal dural enhancement (*yellow arrow*) indicating localized meningitis. (*C*) Further extension of infection/inflammatory process into the cavernous sinuses with enhancement of the walls of the bilateral internal carotid arteries (*circle*) reflecting arteritis as a complication and asymmetric narrowing of the left internal carotid artery (*red arrow*). Focal dural enhancement (*yellow arrow*). (*D, E*) Asymmetric enhancement of the cavernous sinuses, circumferential carotid wall enhancement bilaterally, and narrowing of the left internal carotid artery (*red arrows*). (*F*) Increased signal on DWI signify extension of infection/inflammation into the bilateral cavernous sinuses (*circle*).

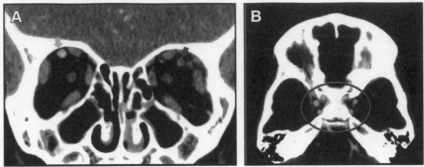

Fig. 8. Contemporaneous orbital CT demonstrates much less dramatic infection and inflammatory changes in the left orbit (*A*) with unremarkable appearance of the bilateral cavernous sinuses (*circle*) (*B*). There is thrombosis of the left superior ophthalmic vein (*red arrow*), as evidenced by its asymmetric lack of contrast enhancement as compared with its normal counterpart (*blue arrow*). This illustrates the superior diagnostic capability of MRI (over CT) in defining the extent of disease and identifying important anatomic structures involved, such as vessels. The extent of disease and involvement vital structures was clearly underestimated on CT. The information provided by MRI was crucial and prompted a more aggressive treatment and better outcome.

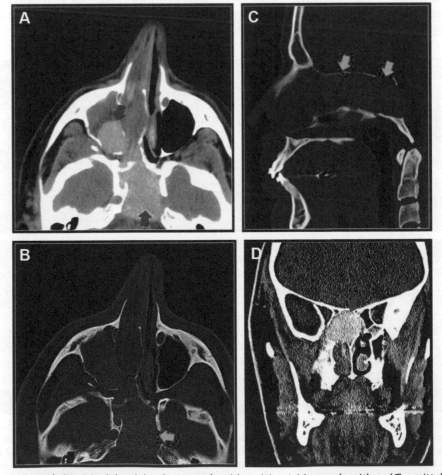

Fig. 9. Allergic fungal sinusitis: (*A*) axial soft tissue algorithm, (*B*) axial bone algorithm, (*C*) sagittal bone algorithm, (*D*) coronal soft tissue algorithm: expansile opacification of the right-sided sinonasal cavities with extensive bony remodeling/erosions (*blue arrow*). There are hyperdense materials (*arrows*) in the right sphenoid and maxillary sinuses (*red arrows*). CT typically shows material of increased attenuation causing opacification and expansion of the sinuses with bony remodeling/erosion. The increased attenuation of AFS is ascribed to the combined effects of heavy metals, such as iron, manganese, and calcium, as well as inspissated mucosal secretions.

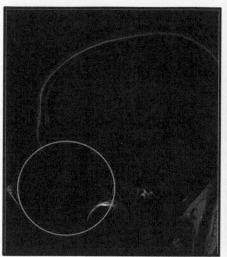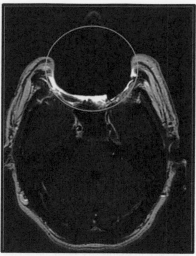

Fig. 10. MRI of allergic fungal sinusitis. MRI demonstrates loss of signal "black-hole" phenomenon (*blue circles*) in the paranasal sinuses. MRI is useful in detecting heavy metals concentrated by fungal elements. Loss of signal is attributed to elevated concentrations of various metals from the fungal organisms, such as manganese, iron, and magnesium, as well as to a high protein and low free-water content of the allergic mucin.

MRI may complement CT (**Fig. 9**) in the diagnosis of chronic sinus conditions such as allergic fungal sinusitis. Low signal intensity or signal void on T2-weighted images is characteristic of allergic fungal sinusitis (**Fig. 10**). This signal void is attributed to high concentrations of various metals, such as iron, magnesium, and manganese concentrated by fungal organisms. This is also

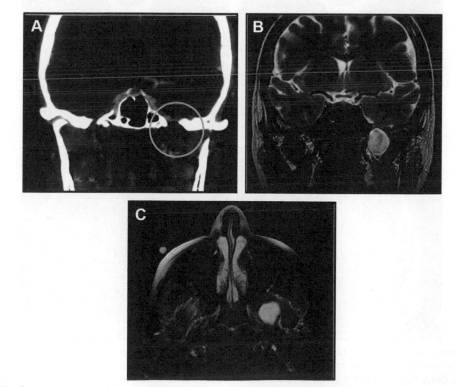

Fig. 11. V3 schwannoma: (*A*) Coronal postcontrast CT, asymmetric expansion of the left foramen ovale with a vague soft mass (*circle*). (*B*) Ovoid T2 hyperintense mass expanding the left foramen ovale. (*C*) Axial postcontrast axial MRI shows enhancement, typical of a nerve sheath tumor. An extracranial meningioma may have a similar appearance.

related to a high protein and a low free-water content of the allergic mucin.[24]

Skull Base and Temporal Bones

In skull base conditions, both MRI and CT may be required to address all clinical and management issues. MR and CT imaging are both important to diagnose trigeminal schwannomas accurately. MRI provides better depiction of the cranial nerves, whereas CT best evaluates the skull base foramina through which the cranial nerves exit (**Fig. 11**).[25,26] In the diagnosis of lesions such as encephalocele, MRI is advantageous because of its excellent soft tissue contrast and multiplanar capability, accurately depicting brain tissue in an aberrant location (**Fig. 12**).

MRI is the primary imaging modality for evaluating the nonosseous components of the temporal bone region.[1,27] In the postoperative setting, MRI is important in the diagnosis of recurrent cholesteatoma. Non-echo planar diffusion-weighted imaging (DWI) increases the sensitivity of conventional MRI on even smaller (ie, less than 5 mm) recurrent cholesteatomas (**Fig. 13**).[28] In the absence of MRI findings indicative of the diagnosis, "second look" surgery may be avoided. Cholesterol granulomas of the petrous apex are expansile, cystic lesions containing cholesterol crystals surrounded by foreign body giant cells, fibrous tissue reaction, and chronic inflammation. These lesions are hyperintense (bright) on T1-weighted sequences (**Fig. 14**).[28]

Vascular Lesions

MRI/magnetic resonance angiography (MRA) is the most valuable noninvasive modality for the classification of vascular anomalies because it accurately demonstrates their location and their anatomic relationship to adjacent structures.[28] Recent advances in MRI have enabled the

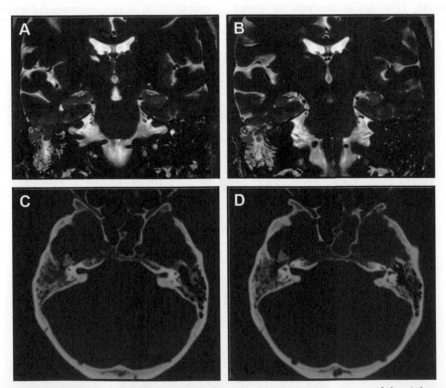

Fig. 12. Meningoencephalocele: (*A, B*) Coronal T2-weighted sequences show portions of the right temporal lobe parenchyma herniating into the mastoid air cells (*red arrows*). (*C, D*) Axial noncontrast CT with bone algorithm depicting a bony defect in the tegmen tympani (*blue arrow heads*), that allowed brain tissue to herniate into the mastoid. An illustration of the multiplanar advantage of MRI combined with its accuracy in defining soft tissues: the correct diagnosis is established by virtue of its accurate depiction of the spatial relationship of anatomic structures. The diagnosis of meningoencephalocele (ie, identification of brain tissue in an aberrant location) is difficult if not impossible on CT.

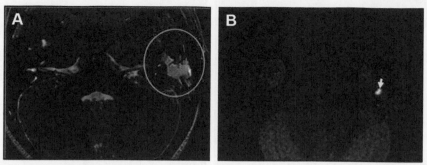

Fig. 13. Recurrent cholesteatoma: (*A*) Postsurgical changes from prior cholesteatoma surgery shown on T2-weighted sequence (*circle*). (*B*) Increased signal in the anterior aspect of the mastoidectomy cavity (*arrow*) on DWI, consistent with recurrent cholesteatoma. In the postoperative setting, MRI is important in the diagnosis of recurrent cholesteatoma. Non-echo planar DWI increases the sensitivity of conventional MRI on even smaller (ie, less than 5 mm) recurrent cholesteatomas, as depicted in this case. "Second-look" surgery may be avoided in the absence of MRI findings.

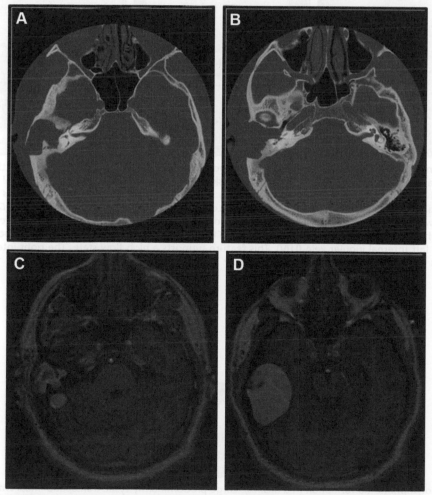

Fig. 14. Petrous apex cholesterol granuloma: (*A, B*) Axial noncontrast CT with bone algorithm shows a lytic expansile process in the right petrous apex. (*C, D*) Axial T1-weighted images with elevated T1 signal corresponding to the expansile lesion. The expansile nature of the lesion and T1 hyperintense signal are typical MRI features of cholesterol granuloma. (*Courtesy of* Eliana E. Bonfante-Mejia, MD, University of Texas Health Science Center, Houston, TX.)

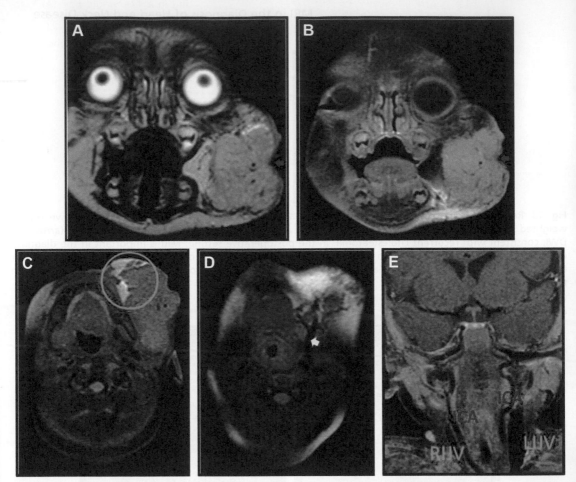

Fig. 15. Infantile hemangioma: (*A*) Coronal T2-weighted MRI, large, lobulated soft tissue mass in the left facial region with a suggestion of ulceration of the overlying skin (*red arrow*, also shown in *B*). (*B*) Coronal postcontrast T1-weighted MRI shows avid enhancement of the mass. (*C*) Axial T1-weighted MRI revealing areas of increased signal within the mass representing methemoglobin, consistent with hemorrhage (*blue circle*). (*D*) Axial non-contrast T1-weighted MRI shows tubular, branching flow-void representing an arterial feeder (*yellow arrow*), indicating a high-flow lesion. (*E*) Coronal noncontrast T1-weighted MR sequence depicting asymmetric enlargement of the left internal jugular vein (LIJV). This feature supports a high-flow state. The right internal jugular vein (RIJV) is normal sized. ICA, internal carotid artery.

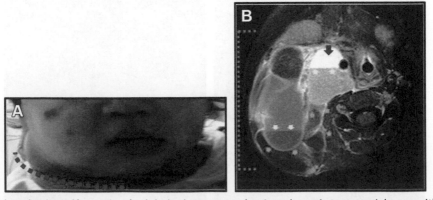

Fig. 16. Venolymphatic malformation (red dashes): Large predominantly cystic transspatial mass with enhancing components and internal fluid-fluid levels. (*A*) Compressible, asymmetric enlargement of the right neck with maroon-red discoloration. (*B*) Fluid-fluid levels (*yellow arrows*), enhancing septae (*blue arrows*), and focal area of increased T1 signal reflecting methemoglobin and recent hemorrhage (*red arrow*). Note the absence of perilesional edema (*dotted bracket*). (*Courtesy of* Megan Kalambo, MD, University of Texas Health Science Center, Houston, TX.)

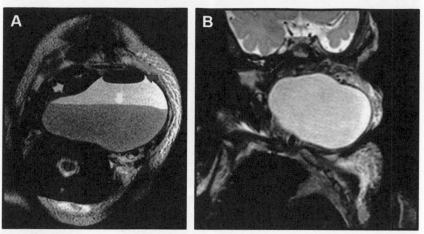

Fig. 17. Enteric duplication cyst in a neonate with rapidly enlarging neck mass and respiratory distress: (*A, B*) T2-weighted MRI shows a very large cyst with substantial mass effect (note anterolateral displacement of upper airway, *blue arrow*). Fluid-fluid level (*yellow arrow*) and gas in the antidependent portion of the cyst (*red arrow*). The presence of gas raised the question of fistulization of the cyst with the upper airway or esophagus. Excision confirmed an enteric duplication cyst with esophageal fistulization. In retrospect, rapid enlargement of the cyst may have been caused or exacerbated by feeding, given the presence of fistula.

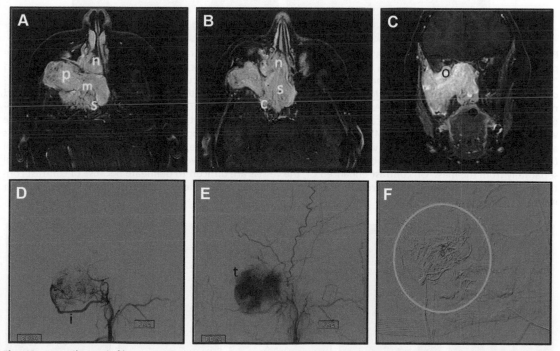

Fig. 18. Juvenile angiofibroma: (*A*) Axial T1 postcontrast MRI: hypervascular tumor expanding the pterygopalatine fossa (p) extending into the adjacent masticator space (m) through the expanded pterygomaxillary fissure and into the nasal cavity (n) through a widened sphenopalatine foramen. Posteriorly, the tumor extends into the skull base (s). (*B*) Axial postcontrast MRI: skull base and intracranial extension of the tumor, with involvement of the cavernous sinus, abutting the internal carotid artery (*arrow*). (*C*) Coronal postcontrast MRI: further depiction of the extent of the tumor occupying the nasal cavity/nasopharynx with orbital invasion (o). (*D, E*) Conventional angiographic correlation, hypervascular mass predominantly fed by branches of the internal maxillary artery (i), with tumor staining (t). (*F*) Onyx cast (*circle*) after endovascular embolization and denudation of the mass.

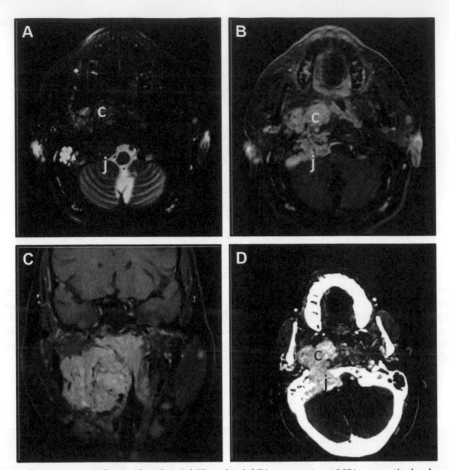

Fig. 19. Jugular fossa paraganglioma: (*A*, *B*) Axial T2 and axial T1 postcontrast MRI, respectively, show a large hypervascular mass in the jugular fossa (j) extending into the carotid space (c). Multiple areas of signal void (called "flow-voids") represent vessels (*red arrows* in *A*, *B*), indicating a highly vascular mass. Note vessel encasement (*circle* in *B*). (*C*) Coronal T1 postcontrast MRI (C) shows the bulk of the mass in the carotid space, with mass-effect and narrowing of the upper airway. (*D*) Axial postcontrast CT shows similar findings with the mass expanding the jugular fossa and extending into the carotid space (C). Vascular encasement is difficult to appreciate because the vessels are obscured by the mass. MRI defines the extent and morphology (including vascularity) of the mass and establishes its relationship with vital structures (ie, vessels). In this case, MRI completely surrounds the vessel (represented by a "flow-void"), reflecting vascular encasement. The flow-void allowed visualization of the vessel separately from the mass. On contrast-enhanced CT, the vessels are difficult to delineate because of contrast contained in the lumen, blending imperceptibly with the background of avid enhancement in this hypervascular mass.

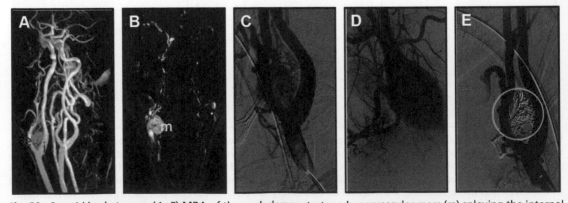

Fig. 20. Carotid body tumor: (*A*, *B*) MRA of the neck demonstrates a hypervascular mass (m) splaying the internal (i) and external (e) carotid arteries characteristic of carotid body tumor. (*C*, *D*) Conventional angiogram confirming the findings on MRA. (*E*) Embolic cast (Onyx) after endovascular treatment (*circle*). This case exemplifies how MRI can characterize vascular lesions with anatomic and flow information.

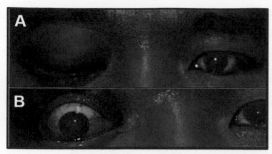

Fig. 21. A 38-year-old Asian man with a history of a motor vehicle collision, suffering a blunt force trauma to the eye resulting in orbital fractures. Repair of the orbital wall fracture was undertaken. (*A*) The patient continues to manifest with complete blepharoptosis and exophthalmos and ophthalmoplegia of the right globe. (*B*) Congestion of the right globe with dilated episcleral and conjunctival vessels. (*Courtesy of* Marc Criden, MD and He Kim Joon, MD, Department of Ophthalmology and Visual Science, University of Texas Medical School, Houston, TX.)

acquisition of dynamic (or time-resolved) angiographic data sets with high spatial and temporal resolution.[29–32] The unique value of MR digital subtraction angiography is its ability to show the passage of a bolus of contrast material through the abnormality in a manner identical to that of conventional angiography. High-flow lesions show rapid contrast enhancement during the early arterial phase and may show enlarged vessels and pathologic arteriovenous shunting with early venous filling. A high-flow lesion is shown in **Fig. 15**. Low-flow lesions, such as venous malformations, may show less dramatic contrast

enhancement on routine MRIs; however, most importantly, the lesions do not show early opacification on MR digital subtraction angiograms. Such lesions show either no vascularity on MR digital subtraction angiograms or appear during the venous phase.[29] MRI is useful in establishing long-term management strategy and in the evaluation of treatment success.[28]

MRI is the cross-sectional imaging of choice in the neck in the pediatric population, because of concerns about radiation exposure with CT.[28,33] MRI is desirable in evaluating soft tissues, transspatial lesions, vascular conditions, and other congenital anomalies.[29,34–37] Examples of such lesions include venolymphatic malformation and duplications cysts (see **Fig. 15**; **Fig. 16**). Although uncommon, foregut duplication cysts (example on **Fig. 17**) of the head and neck should be considered in the differential diagnosis of cystic head and neck lesions.[38]

MRI is useful for the delineation of intracranial extension of juvenile angiofibroma (formerly known as juvenile nasopharyngeal angiofibroma) (**Fig. 18**).[39]

The typical angiographic appearance of a paraganglioma is that of a hypervascular mass with enlarged feeding arteries, intense tumor blush, and early draining veins.[34] Multiple serpentine and punctate areas of signal void (flow-void) characterize the typical paraganglioma with all MR sequences (**Fig. 19**). Although not diagnostic, the classic "salt-and-pepper" appearance of paraganglioma has been described, with the "pepper" component representing multiple areas of signal void and the "salt" as hyperintense (bright) signal because of slow flow and/or hemorrhage.[40] Carotid body tumors typically cause splaying of the

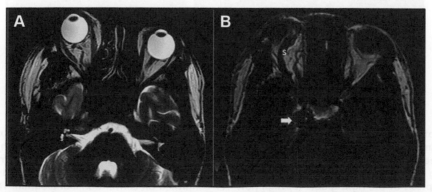

Fig. 22. Conventional MRI in carotid-cavernous sinus fistula (CCF): (*A*) T2-weighted MRI shows proptosis of the right globe. (*B*) Abnormal flow-voids (*arrow*) in the right cavernous sinus region and dilated right superior ophthalmic vein (S) on T1-weighted imaging.

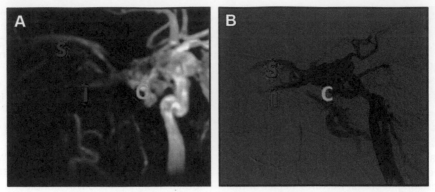

Fig. 23. MRA (*A*) shows excellent correlation with conventional angiogram (*B*) in CCF. CCF, carotid-cavernous sinus fistula (C). Note dilated superior (S) and inferior (I) ophthalmic veins.

external and internal carotid arteries (**Fig. 20**). The most common feeding vessels to any head and neck paraganglioma are the ascending pharyngeal artery (via the musculospinal artery) and the ascending cervical artery.[40]

MRA is indicated to demonstrate the presence, nature, and extent of injury to the cervicocerebral vessels.[28] In the setting of trauma, noninvasive tests such as 3-dimensional time-of-flight MRA and/or computed tomographic angiography (CTA) proved to be useful in the noninvasive diagnosis of carotid-cavernous sinus fistula (**Figs. 21–24**) before an invasive digital subtraction angiography was undertaken. MRA and/or CTA source images provided useful information not obtainable on conventional angiogram in some cases.[41]

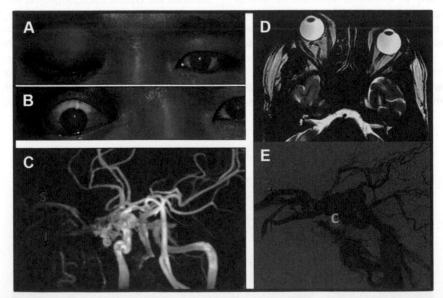

Fig. 24. Carotid-cavernous sinus fistula (CCF): summary of findings. (*A*) Complete blepharoptosis, exophthalmos, and ophthalmoplegia of the right globe. (*B*) Right globe congestion with dilated episcleral and conjunctival vessels. (*C*) Three dimensional time-of-flight MRA with abnormal flow-related signal in the right cavernous sinus (C) representing CCF; also with dilated superior (S) and inferior (I) ophthalmic veins. (*D*) T2-weighted MRI demonstrating proptosis of the right globe. (*E*) High-flow CCF confirmed on conventional angiogram. This case illustrates an excellent correlation between a noninvasive diagnostic modality (MRI/MRA) in the setting of vascular trauma. The information provided by a noninvasive diagnostic test offered by MRI/MRA is important in planning endovascular therapeutic approach.

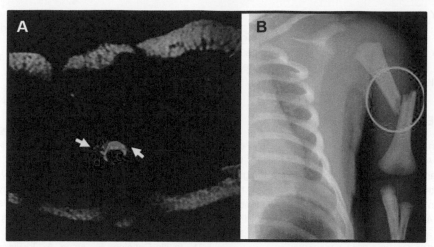

Fig. 25. Brachial plexus - traumatic pseudomeningocele: (*A*) Axial T2-weighed sequence shows asymmetric enlargement of the nerve root sleeves (*yellow arrows*), with a pseudomeningocele on the right. This is an example of a birth injury to the brachial plexus acquired during a difficult delivery. (*B*) Fracture of the left humerus in the same patient (*circle*). c, lower cervical cord; d, dorsal root; v, ventral root.

Brachial Plexus

MRI is valuable in the evaluation of brachial plexus injuries, particularly in neonates.[42,43] Stretching, also called "neuropraxia," injuries are commonly seen in neonates, particularly after breech deliveries with shoulder dystocia.[43–45]

The presence of traumatic pseudomeningocele and the absence of roots are important signs of injury.[42] Nerve root avulsion commonly occurs without a meningocele, and a meningocele occasionally exists without nerve root avulsion.[46] Pseudomeningoceles appear as a tear in the meningeal sheath that surrounds the nerve roots. Because of fluid filling the pseudomeningocele, they are easily identifiable on T2-weighted MRIs (**Fig. 25**).[43]

MRI is useful the evaluation of masses in the brachial plexus in adults. Malignant peripheral nerve sheath tumors are less common (**Fig. 26**). These tumors are frequently large (exceeding 5 cm) and present with worsening pain or new neurologic deficits. Enhancement and topography are depicted by current MRI techniques, although imaging findings may not accurately predict benignity of the lesion. More advanced techniques like diffusion tensor imaging will likely play a role in the future, in understanding the behavior of these lesions by providing functional insight.[47]

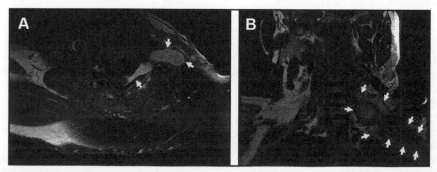

Fig. 26. Brachial plexus: (*A, B*) Malignant peripheral nerve sheath tumor (neurofibrosarcoma): images show a mass-like, irregular enlargement of the left brachial plexus (*arrows*). (*Courtesy of* Scott Benjamin Serlin, MD, University of Texas Health Science Center, Houston, TX.)

SUMMARY

This article has provided illustrative cases high-lighting the value and important applications of MRI in the diagnosis and management of head and neck disease.

REFERENCES

1. American College of Radiology Appropriateness Criteria. ACR-ASNR-SPR Practice Guideline for the Performance of Magnetic Resonance Imaging (MRI) of the Head and Neck. Revised 2012 (Res. 19).
2. American College of Radiology Appropriateness Criteria. ACR-ASNR-SPR Practice Guideline for Performing and Interpreting Magnetic Resonance Imaging (MRI). Revised 2011 (Res. 19).
3. American College of Radiology Glossary of MRI Terms.
4. Abdel Razek A, King A. MRI and CT of nasopharyngeal carcinoma. AJR Am J Roentgenol 2012;198:11–8.
5. King A, Bhatia KS. Magnetic resonance imaging staging of nasopharyngeal carcinoma in the head and neck. World J Radiol 2010;2:159–65.
6. Vandevyver V, Lemmerling M, Van Hecke W, et al. MRI findings of the normal and diseased trigeminal nerve ganglion and branches: a pictorial review. JBR–BTR 2007;90:272–7.
7. Curtin HD, Williams RW, Johnson J. CT of perineural tumor extension: pterygopalatine fossa. AJNR Am J Neuroradiol 1984;5:731–7.
8. Nemzek R, Hecht S, Gandour-Edwards R, et al. Perineural spread of head and neck tumors: how accurate is MR imaging? AJNR Am J Neuroradiol 1998;19:701–6.
9. Catalano PJ, Sen C, Biller HF. Cranial neuropathy secondary to perineural spread of cutaneous malignancies. Am J Otol 1995;16:772–7.
10. Donald P. Skull base surgery. Otolaryngol Head Neck Surg 1992;106:10–1.
11. Sham JS, Cheung YK, Choy D, et al. Cranial nerve involvement and base of skull erosion in nasopharyngeal carcinoma. Cancer 1991;68:422–6.
12. Ikeda K, Katoh T, Ha-Kawa SK, et al. The usefulness of MR in establishing the diagnosis of parotid pleomorphic adenoma. AJNR Am J Neuroradiol 1996;17:555–9.
13. Som PM, Biller HF. High-grade malignancies of parotid gland: identification with MR imaging. Radiology 1989;173:823–6.
14. Swartz JD, Rothman MI, Marlowe FI, et al. MR imaging of parotid mass lesions: attempts at histopathologic differentiation. J Comput Assist Tomogr 1989;13:789–96.
15. Freling NJ, Molenaar WM, Vermey A, et al. Malignant parotid tumors: clinical use of MR imaging and histological correlation. Radiology 1992;185:691–6.
16. Schalakman BN, Yousem DM. MR of intraparotid masses. AJNR Am J Neuroradiol 1993;14:1173–80.
17. Kurabayashi T, Ida M, Yasumoto M, et al. MRI of ranulas. Neuroradiology 2000;42:917–22.
18. Barnes PD, Robson CD, Robertson RL, et al. Pediatric orbital and visual pathway lesions. Neuroimaging Clin N Am 1996;6:179–98.
19. Ortiz O, Flores RA. Clinical and radiologic evaluation of optic pathway lesions. Semin Ultrasound CT MR 1998;19:225–39.
20. Zimmerman RA, Bilaniuk LT, Savino PJ. Chapter 11: visual pathways: embryology, anatomy and pathology. In: Som PM, Curtin HD, editors. Head and neck imaging. 4th edition. Philadelphia: Mosby; 2003. p. 735–82.
21. Tovilla-Canales JL, Nava A, Tovilla y Pomar JL. Orbital and periorbital infections. Curr Opin Ophthalmol 2001;12:335–41.
22. Kapur R, Sepahdari AR, Mafee MF, et al. MR imaging of orbital inflammatory syndrome, orbital cellulitis, and orbital lymphoid lesions: the role of diffusion-weighted imaging. AJNR Am J Neuroradiol 2009;30(1):64–70.
23. Sepahdari AR, Aakalu VK, Kapur R, et al. MRI of orbital cellulitis and orbital abscess: the role of diffusion-weighted imaging. AJR Am J Roentgenol 2009;193(3):W244–50.
24. Aribandi M, McCoy VA, Bazan C. Imaging features of invasive and non-invasive fungal sinusitis: a review. Radiographics 2007;27:1283–96.
25. Abdel Razek A, Castillo M. Imaging lesions of the cavernous sinus. AJNR Am J Neuroradiol 2009;30:444–52.
26. Mehra S, Garga UC, Suresh. Radiological imaging in trigeminal nerve schwannoma: a case report and review of literature. JIMSA 2013;26:2.
27. Chakeres DW. Augustyn. Chapter 20: temporal bone: imaging anatomy. In: Som PM, Curtin HD, editors. Head and neck imaging. 4th edition. Philadelphia: Mosby; 2003. p. 1095–108.
28. Barátha K, Huberb A, Stämpflid P, et al. Neuroradiology of cholesteatomas. AJNR Am J Neuroradiol 2011;32:221–9.
29. American College of Radiology Appropriateness Criteria. ACR-ASNR-SNIS-SPR Practice Guideline for the Performance of Magnetic Resonance Imaging (MRI) of the Head and Neck. Revised 2010 (Res. 21).
30. Chooi WK, Woodhouse N, Coley SC, et al. Pediatric head and neck lesions: assessment of vascularity by MR digital subtraction angiography. AJNR Am J Neuroradiol 2004;25:1251–5.
31. Strecker R, Scheffler K, Klisch J, et al. Fast functional MRA using time-resolved projection MR angiography with correlation analysis. Magn Reson Med 2000;43:303–9.

32. Hennig J, Scheffler K, Laubenberger J, et al. Time-resolved projection angiography after bolus injection of contrast agent. Magn Reson Med 1997;37: 341–5.

33. Wang Y, Johnston DL, Breen JF, et al. Dynamic MR digital subtraction angiography using contrast enhancement, fast data acquisition, and complex subtraction. Magn Reson Med 1996;36:551–6.

34. Meuwly JY, Lepori D, Theumann N, et al. Multimodality imaging evaluation of the pediatric neck: techniques and spectrum of findings. Radiographics 2005;25:931–48.

35. Flors L, Leiva-Salinas C, Maged I, et al. MR imaging of soft-tissue vascular malformations: diagnosis, classification, and therapy follow-up. Radiographics 2011;31:1321–40.

36. Dubois J. Vascular anomalies: what a radiologist needs to know. Pediatr Radiol 2010;40:895–905.

37. Zadvinskis DP, Benson MT, Kerr HH, et al. Congenital malformations of the cervicothoracic lymphatic system: embryology and pathogenesis. Radiographics 1992;12:1175–89.

38. Kieran SM, Robson CD, Nosé V, et al. Foregut duplication cysts in the head and neck: presentation, diagnosis, and management. Arch Otolaryngol Head Neck Surg 2010;136:8.

39. Riascos R, et al. Imaging and anatomic features of juvenile angiofibroma. Neurographics 2011;1(2): 84–9.

40. Rao A, Koeller K, Adair C. Paragangliomas of the head and neck: radiologic-pathologic correlation. Radiographics 1999;19:1605–32.

41. Chi-Chang C, Chang PC, Shy CG, et al. CT angiography and MR angiography in the evaluation of carotid cavernous sinus fistula prior to embolization: a comparison of techniques. AJNR Am J Neuroradiol 2005;26:2349–56.

42. Takeharu Yoshikawa T, Hayashi N, Yamamoto S. Brachial plexus injury: clinical manifestations, conventional imaging findings, and the latest imaging techniques. Radiographics 2006;26: S133–43.

43. Castillo M. Imaging the anatomy of the brachial plexus: review and self-assessment module. AJR Am J Roentgenol 2005;185:S196–204.

44. Guha A, Graham B, Kline DG, et al. Brachial plexus injuries. In: Wilkins RH, Rengachary SS, editors. Neurosurgery. 2nd edition. New York: McGraw-Hill; 1996. p. 3121–34.

45. Piatt JH. Birth injuries of the brachial plexus. Pediatr Clin North Am 2004;51:421–40.

46. Ochi M, Ikuta Y, Watanabe M, et al. The diagnostic value of MRI in traumatic brachial plexus injury. J Hand Surg Br 1994;19:55–9.

47. Chhabra A, Thawait G, Soldatos T, et al. High-resolution 3T MR neurography of the brachial plexus and its branches, with emphasis on 3D imaging. AJNR Am J Neuroradiol 2013;34:486–97.

Index

Note: Page numbers of article titles are in **boldface** type.

Oral Maxillofacial Surg Clin N Am 26 (2014) 271–275
http://dx.doi.org/10.1016/S1042-3699(14)00022-3
1042-3699/14/$ – see front matter © 2014 Elsevier Inc. All rights reserved.

Moving?

Make sure your subscription moves with you!

To notify us of your new address, find your **Clinics Account Number** (located on your mailing label above your name), and contact customer service at:

Email: journalscustomerservice-usa@elsevier.com

800-654-2452 (subscribers in the U.S. & Canada)
314-447-8871 (subscribers outside of the U.S. & Canada)

Fax number: 314-447-8029

Elsevier Health Sciences Division
Subscription Customer Service
3251 Riverport Lane
Maryland Heights, MO 63043

*To ensure uninterrupted delivery of your subscription, please notify us at least 4 weeks in advance of move.

Moving?

Make sure your subscription moves with you!

To notify us of your new address, find your **Clinics Account Number** (located on your mailing label above your name), and contact customer service at:

Email: journalscustomerservice-usa@elsevier.com

800-654-2452 (subscribers in the U.S. & Canada)
314-447-8871 (subscribers outside of the U.S. & Canada)

Fax number: 314-447-8029

Elsevier Health Sciences Division
Subscription Customer Service
3251 Riverport Lane
Maryland Heights, MO 63043

Printed and bound by CPI Group (UK) Ltd, Croydon, CR0 4YY

03/10/2024

01040377-0012